MW01222279

Creating a Miracle Child With Yoga

The Practical and Complete Guide for Expectant Parents

Veena S. Gandhi, M.D., FACOG

Dear Dyan and Dave
with Love.
Veena S. Gandhi
~ 2013 ~

Creating a Miracle Child with Yoga
The Practical and Complete Guide for Expectant Parents

Copyright © 2012 Veena S. Gandhi, M.D.

All rights reserved. No part of this book may be used or reproduced by any means, graphic, electronic, or mechanical, including photocopying, recording, taping or by any information storage retrieval system without the written permission of the publisher except in the case of brief quotations embodied in critical articles and reviews.

ISBN: 978-1-4582-0299-4 (hbk)

ISBN: 978-1-4582-0298-7 (sc)

ISBN: 978-1-4582-0716-6 (e)

Library of Congress Control Number: 2012905960

Abbott Press books may be ordered through booksellers or by contacting:

Abbott Press
1663 Liberty Drive
Bloomington, IN 47403
www.abbottpress.com
Phone: 1-866-697-5310

Because of the dynamic nature of the Internet, any web addresses or links contained in this book may have changed since publication and may no longer be valid. The views expressed in this work are solely those of the author and do not necessarily reflect the views of the publisher, and the publisher hereby disclaims any responsibility for them.

Any people depicted in stock imagery provided by Thinkstock are models, and such images are being used for illustrative purposes only.

Certain stock imagery © Thinkstock.

Printed in the United States of America

Abbott Press rev. date: 11/16/2012

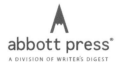

abbott press®
A DIVISION OF WRITER'S DIGEST

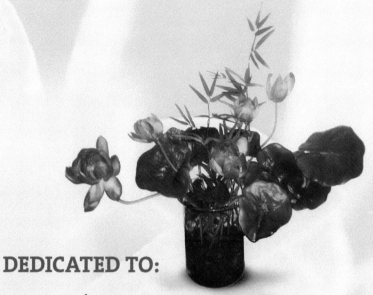

DEDICATED TO:

My parents who with great energy, love, simplicity, and wisdom raised me **&** *all the expectant parents who hope to create a "miracle child."*

Exercise during pregnancy can help prepare you for labor and childbirth. Exercising afterward can help get you back in shape.

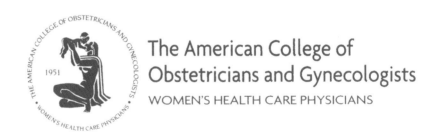

The American College of
Obstetricians and Gynecologists
WOMEN'S HEALTH CARE PHYSICIANS

Contents

Medical Disclaimer

Please consult your physician prior to participation in any yoga program. The instructions and advice presented are not intended as a substitute for medical care. In general, modified yoga for pregnancy is very safe since it is done with conscious breathing and mindfulness. Please make sure that you learn from a well-trained certified yoga teacher.

According to the American College of OB/GYN, pregnant women can continue to exercise and derive the health benefits from participating in mild to moderate intensity exercise routines.

Yoga should be done on a regular basis. Properly done yoga postures and yogic breathing should not lead to shortness of breath. If shortness of breath occurs, the postures and breathing should be slowed and shortened. Relaxation poses bring lots of restful energy.

Postures lying on the back should be avoided after the late second trimester. In general, inversion postures are to be avoided or modified. The balancing poses may be difficult during pregnancy, especially in the later part of the second and third trimesters, so one should avoid or modify them.

Adequate and proper diet and hydration during pregnancy is very essential.

Yoga should be continued during the postpartum period and later on with the baby. The infant can also be exposed to yoga right from the early months.

Yoga helps in conditions like gestational diabetes and pregnancy-induced hypertension, especially relaxation poses on the left lateral side, "shavasana". Yoga has also been found to help in intrauterine growth retardation (www.svyasa.org).

Please do not do yoga if you have the following conditions: preterm rupture of membranes, preterm labor during a prior or current pregnancy, incompetent cervix/cerclage (sutures on mouth of the uterus to prevent miscarriage and preterm labor), or persistent first, second, or third trimester bleeding.

Women with certain other medical conditions like cardiac, pulmonary, skeletal, or vascular diseases should be evaluated very carefully by their obstetrician before starting to practice yoga.

If the following symptoms occur: sudden sharp pain, nausea or vomiting, faintness or dizziness, or irregularity of heartbeat, stop and lie on your left side. If symptoms persist after a few minutes, call your physician.

Because yogic exercises are done slowly, with conscious breathing and awareness, to the best of your capacity, they are very safe. Enjoy. If yoga is done incorrectly and/or differently than instructed in this book, the author does not assume responsibility.

Forward

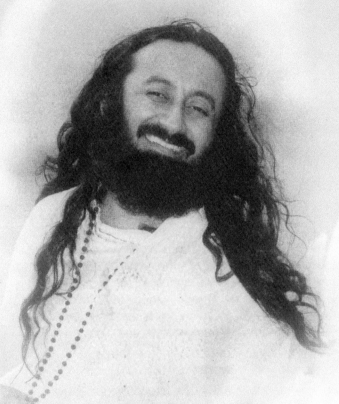

At a time when women are emerging into new roles, and choosing motherhood later in their lives well into their forties, this book by Dr. Veena S. Gandhi comes as a refreshing reprieve and comfort, providing amazing insight into one of the most important periods in a woman's life. It is said that" "Mother is the first Guru". If that is true, this book is a celebration for all mothers-to-be.

In this book you will find an easy and comprehensive introduction to yoga where its goal is described as – "to be harmonious". If pregnancy is indeed the highest creative period in a woman's life, then through yoga's multi-system balancing approach this book shines light on giving birth to a healthy, balanced and harmonious soul.

The book's step-by-step approach and easy flow guides you through the various states of pregnancy: pre-conception, labor, and post-partum, each stage supported by yoga postures (asanas), yogic breathing (pranayamas), a yogic diet, as well as practical wisdom to live by for the expectant couple. Thus, creating a loving receptacle for the new baby to arrive and thrive in love and harmony.

Dr. Veena S. Gandhi blends her forty years of OB/GYN experience and yoga knowledge in this amazing work, providing a unique perspective for expectant mothers to bring a miracle baby into this world.

I am sure, all readers will find much upon these pages to guide, comfort and inspire them during this happy yet stressful time in their life.

Sri Sri Ravi Shanker
President and Founder -
Art of Living (Worldwide)
www.artofliving.org

Blessings

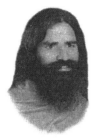 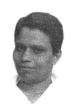

!! ॐ !!

पतंजलि योगपीठ (ट्रस्ट)

द्वारा संचालित

पतंजलि योग समिति

मुख्यालय : महर्षि दयानन्द ग्राम, दिल्ली–हरिद्वार राष्ट्रीय राजमार्ग, निकट बहादराबाद, हरिद्वार – 249402, उत्तरांखण्ड, भारत

The present day society is at a crossroads; ever increasing violence, terrorism, drugs, divorces and broken families compel us to think about how to stop these vulgarities and create a new society with love, harmony and peace. This should start right from intra-uterine life.

"Creating a miracle child with yoga," the complete and practical guide for the expectant parents, provides a great insight in this field. The role of yoga during planning of pregnancy, during pregnancy and after the delivery brings out the great results. The newborn is blessed with not only good physical health, but also with a great mind and spirit.

This science of yoga is very well proven and respected in the eastern part of the world but it is not as much known in the western world. The author of this book, Dr. Veena S. Gandhi has practiced obstetrics and gynecology in U.S.A. for more that 30 years and is fully confident that this book will tremendously help all the expectant parents.

My blessings and best wishes for this book. May we create a great future generation.

With Love

Swami Ramdevji
Patanjali Yog Peeth,
Haridwar, India

Preface

Yoga is one of the six classical systems of philosophies in India. Ayurveda embraces Sankhya philosophy, which is closely allied with the philosophies of yoga. Patanjali is considered the founder of yoga philosophy, was the first enlightened master to write the yoga sutras in a scientific, almost mathematical language. He rejuvenated yoga into a practice and made it a discipline so that it helps one achieve the four goals of life. Dharma (righteous duty), artha (monetary success), Kama (fulfillment of positive desires) and moksha (enlightenment). Yoga is a timeless, ancient healing art and science that creates physical, mental and spiritual well-being in the life of every human being.

The Sanskrit word "yoga" means "union." It is the union between the lower self and the higher self, guiding one to transcend the individual consciousness into cosmic consciousness (higher consciousness). The practice of yogasanas (yoga postures) and pranayama (breathing exercises) need proper guidance. Although the poses and pranayamas outlined in this book can be practiced safely by most people, it's important to follow Dr. Gandhi's recommendations throughout the book.

Every yoga posture and pranayama has its own unique psycho-physiologic and therapeutic value. Dr. Veena S. Gandhi, M.D., OB/GYN has created a wonderful integration of ancient yoga and modern science. She has been practicing yoga since her early childhood and has been an OB/GYN practitioner for 40 years. Applying yoga therapy with her patients in her practice has led to wonderful success for the health and well-being of her clients and their babies.

This book is her unique integration of yoga and pregnancy. It helps couples achieve a healthy pregnancy and a happy, smooth delivery of their "miracle children". She suggests that both partners perform the yogasanas, pranayama and meditation together. This togetherness will bring love, compassion and proper healthy growth in the fetus. This yoga practice helps to harmonize the partners and develop a loving, happy family environment for the growing child. Dr. Gandhi's approach is very positive, practical and simple, helping families to grow and nourish their daily relationships and make their houses into "happy homes."

Vasant Lad, B.A.M.S., M.A.Sc.
Ayurvedic Physician
Albuquerque, New Mexico

Introduction

The conception and birth of a child is a miracle. It's an experience that is unique and awesome. It is unparalleled in its ability to make us marvel at God's greatest gift. It is the highest and finest creation of cosmic intelligence and cosmic energy found in the entire universe.

For a woman, motherhood is the pinnacle of all experiences. It leads to a unique satisfaction, giving her the finest opportunity to express her highest state of consciousness and vast new energy. For a father, it offers the chance to be truly one with his mate and to give love to the newborn in countless ways.

To create such an intricate manifestation with its full potential, the science of yoga offers the perfect methodology. The path of yoga, which means "union," provides the mapping of creation. To create a miracle child, a couple needs to learn, contemplate, and follow the path of yoga leading to "wholeness." When this "wholeness" is achieved, the couple has successfully merged their physical, mental, and spiritual dimensions to create a "miracle child."

I wrote this book to help couples conceive and deliver their own "miracle" children. My husband and I practiced yoga to deliver our gorgeous boy and girl to the universe. Although they are now grown, their unique ability to give love and to make the world a better place amazes me.

I've also helped countless couples learn yoga to conceive their miracle children and to joyfully deliver them. One memorable patient, Raya Morok*, came to me ready and willing to conceive, but her periods were very irregular, making ovulation difficult. I advised her to attend yoga classes that I was conducting at a local school, along with her husband. They did attend the classes and the outcome was excellent. By participating in my weekly yoga classes, practicing yogic breathing 30 minutes per day, taking her prenatal vitamins, and adopting a yogic diet and lifestyle, Raya's menstrual cycle became more regular in six months. In another four months, she was pregnant.

Overjoyed with the news, the couple continued to follow my advice for creating a "miracle child" through practicing yoga and embracing its spiritual and physical gifts. At 39 weeks, she went into labor, and I delivered a beautiful baby

To create a miracle child, a couple needs to learn, contemplate, and follow the path of yoga leading to "wholeness."

"No teaching or words can convey the value of yoga. It has to be experienced."

boy a few hours later. Best of all, her postpartum time was especially happy. Unlike many new mothers who are exhausted from the labor and the months preceding it, Raya was filled with joy, enthusiasm, and energy. This, I feel, was due to the couple continuing to practice a yogic lifestyle. Her baby boy also had no allergies of any kind and was growing by leaps and bounds.

This "miracle child" is just one of many that have come into the world with yoga's help. For 40 years I've practiced obstetrics and gynecology, first in India and then in the United States. This book is my gift to you, couples that yearn to conceive beautiful children to make the universe a more spiritual and rewarding place.

* Name changed for privacy purposes

Chapter 1: What Is Yoga?

The art and science of yoga has been practiced since time immemorial in India. It is vividly described in detail in "Bhagwat Gita", a scripture written approximately 4000 years ago and subsequently very scientifically analyzed in "Patangali Yoga Sutra" written approximately 2500 years ago. Yoga brings about the positive effects on all planes of human existence: body, mind, intellect and spirit simultaneously. It is the total harmony, outside with the external world and harmony within. The word "yoga" is derived from the Sanskrit root word "Yuj," which means to join, leading to unity and oneness. In spiritual terms it refers to the union of individual to individual consciousness and individual consciousness to universal consciousness, union of lower self to higher self, leading to "bliss." Bliss represents unbounded joy, true knowledge, and absolute truth. The person feels contentment, harmony and total freedom.

In yoga the body is stimulated, stretched, and relaxed to promote exercise to all of the muscle groups of the body. Unlike many other kinds of physical exercises, yoga also works in a subtle way. It exercises the endocrine system; the circulatory system; the central nervous system; the autonomic nervous system; the uro-genital system, the skeleto-muscular system, and the gastrointestinal system. Through yoga's gentle movements with breath and awareness, you can utilize the innate life force within your body and learn how to harness and direct it skillfully.

Yoga is especially good for relieving stress because it helps to channel out negative emotions and mental stress to help feel positive, energetic, and peaceful.

Everyone has experienced these moments at some time or another in their lives—when time stops, place is irrelevant, and people are oblivious, yet there is this unique state of "being" which is beyond all the known perceptions, that is alert, silent, joyful, and harmonious with the cosmic consciousness. This is the depth of yoga.

- When eyes are open but not engaged in seeing the scene
- When ears are open but not engaged in listening
- When the mundane world has disappeared into oblivion this is yoga: total freedom.

The most scientific and well-known book on yoga is the *Yoga Sutras of Patanjali*, originating approximately 2500 years ago in India. Patanjali describes this state as "one which is beyond all the modifications of mind and memory. When that happens, one shines in "self." That is yoga. It releases one from all the superimposed identities, so in true spirit it is deconditioning from the acquired habits to your true self.

It is also very interesting to note that in Taittiriya Upanishad, in "Anand Valli", an important part of ancient Vedic literature, the joy of achieving this state is quantified. Imagine joy obtained by the healthiest, the most beautiful, the richest, young adult as "one unit" of joy, then the joy achieved by the highest yogic state as million times more.

Yoga is the restraint of mental operations. Then the staying of the perceiver in his/her real-self.

Patanjali Yog Sutra 1:2 / 1:3

Truly the joy of yoga is beyond any mundane joys, including riches, great success, or other worlds like heaven. Such is the experience of every successful yoga practitioner. To achieve this state of joy, you need to be persistent, focused with unending devotion, and able to meet all challenges along the way. Yoga is a spark. Once experienced, it never goes out.

Yoga is certainly not postures alone as is often thought. The healthy mind lives in the healthy body, and the healthy spirit lives in the healthy mind. That's why one must keep body and mind, which are temples of the spirit, healthy to achieve the many joys of yoga.

The "body" is kept healthy by achieving a balanced life through engaging in proper activities, proper rest, proper diet, and proper physical exercises. These exercises are known as "asanas," which are postures usually done slowly to an individual's capacity, coordinated with proper breath and united with the mind and spirit called "awareness."

The "mind" is kept healthy by positive thoughts, positive association, and "meditation." The special techniques of breathing, which are part of "Pranayama," help a great deal in calming the mind and discarding anxieties and worries. Pranayama , or breathing techniques are the bridge between the mind and body.

"Meditation" is the culmination of yogic practices. When the mind is brought into a receptive cocoon, a new energy and intuitiveness comes into being. This renewal brings about great transformation and joy. There is a harmony inside and outside.

Restlessness, external hurry, confusion, conflict, contradiction, shakiness, indecisiveness, energy depletion, insecurity, and psychological uncertainty disappear through yoga. The result is clarity of thought, compassion, unselfishness, relaxation, skillful action, and expansiveness of love.

The goal of yoga is to be harmonious. Yoga is a journey within. Desires, fear, and greed plague the mind. Confront them all. Courage, confidence and contentment will flow into you. There are many techniques used to achieve this goal. Since we all know that every human being is unique in his or her genetic makeup and upbringing, there cannot be one technique for all. That's why different techniques are proposed by different teachers.

But you must understand and realize that as you progress in your pursuit of yoga, all techniques merge into one another. In the ultimate stage, there is the same outcome, unity and harmony – within and without.

Friends, for the first time yoga student and readers, this whole concept and the following details may be a little difficult to understand and digest, but for the people with different levels of yogic practices and yogic knowledge, the depth of yoga philosophy is offered here. Please do not get discouraged and be persistent with your theory and practices of yoga to reap the benefits to the fullest.

The goal of yoga is to be harmonious.
Yoga is a journey within.

Yoga is freedom

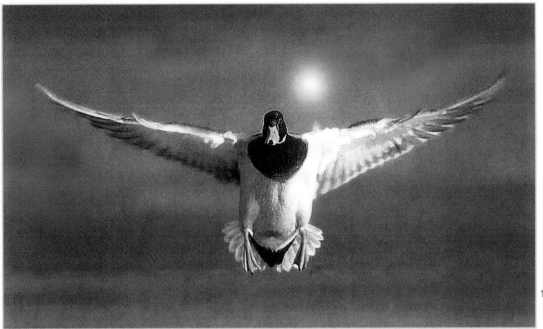

1.1

Yoga balances emotions, leading to equanimity in favorable or unfavorable circumstances.

Yoga is peace

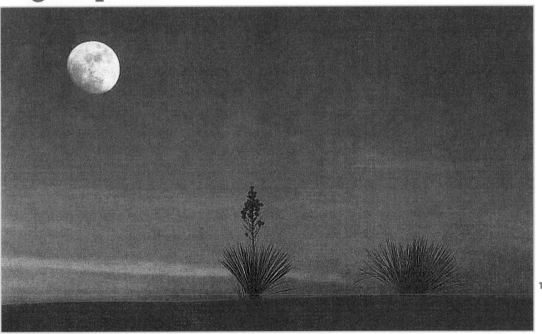

1.2

Yoga reduces stress.

Yoga is joy

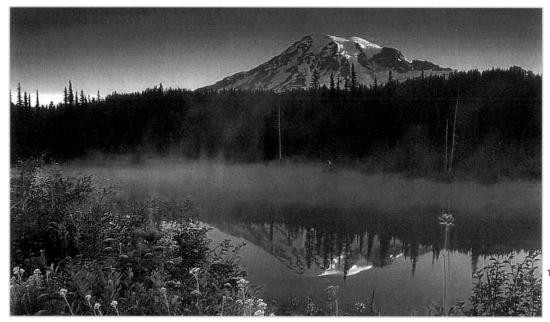

Yoga promotes love for oneself and for others.

Yoga is expansion

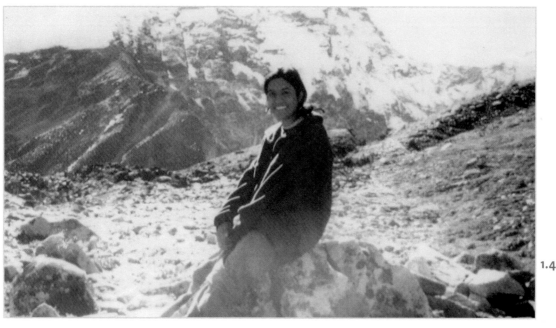

Yoga brings wisdom to help distinguish between real and unreal projections of the cosmos.

The major groups of yoga are:

1. Raja Yoga: Path of mastery over mind

2. Bhakti Yoga: Path of Devotion. "Kirtan" and "Japa", which means chanting repeatedly powerful potentiated words with engrossed mind leading to the higher consciousness. The whole universe is God's creation and so one loves each and every living and non-living thing.

3. Gnana Yoga: Path of knowledge, logical inquiry into "Who am I?" Where will I be after death? What is truly real and what is unreal?

4. Karma Yoga: Path of action. Work diligently, fully, with the best of your capacity, then accept the result that God has blessed you with. Be unattached and surrender all to God.

These four major types of yoga are further expanded into several subtypes.

Major Subtypes of Raja Yoga

• **Hatha Yoga:** Perfected postures with breathing and awareness. The word "Hatha" is Sanskrit syllables "ha" (sun) and "tha" (moon). It is the union of these two. Primarily it deals with the physical body; asanas, pranayama and awareness.

• **Ashtang Yoga of Patanjali:** Eight limb yoga where "samadhi" is the final stage which is a superconscious state. There are many types of samadhis. (See the book *Patanjali Yoga Sutra*)

The eight limbs of Ashtang yoga:

• **Yama:** Truthfulness; nonviolence; continence - chastity (moral sex); not stealing; not collecting more than your basic needs; and not receiving gifts.

• **Niyama:** Contentment; internal and external cleanliness that is cleanliness of thoughts, speech, and actions; self-study; self-restraint; and adoration of God

• **Asana:** Postures for physical fitness that ultimately lead to the ability to sit for a long duration of time for contemplation and meditation

• **Pranayama:** Technique to control "Prana" or vital energy; usually by different types of definitive breathing techniques

• **Pratyahara:** Restraining of the senses & withdrawing from objects of desire

• **Dharana:** Holding and fixing the mind on certain points to the exclusion of all others, that is, concentrating on one object or one thought.

• **Dhyana:** Contemplation on the self or atman (meditation)

• **Samadhi:** State of super-consciousness

The first five limbs are physically oriented, and the last three are mentally oriented.

• **Kundalini Yoga:** Awakening of energy in the spinal column (Sushumna) through meditation. There are seven "chakras." In a simplistic way, chakras are junction of sympathetic and para sympathetic ganglions. These are situated at the crossings of nerves "Ida" and "Pingala" in the back of the body. (for the details about Chakras see the diagram next page).

The Chakras
Flow of energy

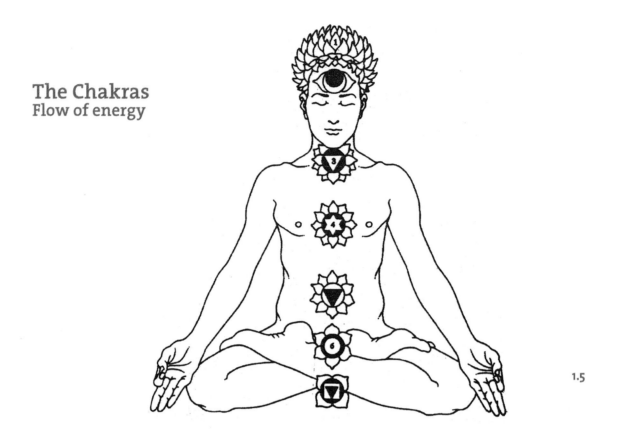

1.5

1. **Head Center**	3. **Throat Center**	5. **Navel Center**	7. **Root Center**
Consciousness-Space	Ether	Fire	Earth
Causal Sound	Sound	Sight	Smell
Causal Prana	Vata	Pita	Kapha
Om	Ham	Ram	Lam
2. **Third Eye**	4. **Heart Center**	6. **Sex Center**	
Mind-Space	Air	Water	
Subtle Sound	Touch	Taste	
Subtle Prana	Vata	Kapha	*Ayurveda and the Mind*
Ksham	Yam	Vam	by Dr. David Frawley

Further detail analysis of these chakras is beyond the scope of this book. Please refer to the above book.

While doing pranayama or meditation, one needs to sit tall for the upward flow of energy through the spine, which in turn affects the mind, intellect, and helps ultimately to unite with consciousness.

There are also some specific named yoga, such as Vini yoga, power yoga, Jeevan Mukti yoga, Vikram yoga, etc. by different yoga teachers. Whatever name for which it is called, the goal is similar or almost the same – yoga is for all, irrespective of religion, nationality or gender.

The Physical/Physiological Benefits of Yoga

- Yoga improves muscle and joint flexibility and endurance.

- Yoga promotes better breathing and increases hemoglobin, thereby boosting its oxygen content, which leads to healthier and stronger tissues.

- Yoga increases circulation to the distant tissues. It decreases the formation of varicose veins.

- Yoga rids the body of all toxins. It improves digestion and regularity.

- Yoga balances the endocrine system and hormones.

- Yoga creates balance between the sympathetic and parasympathetic autonomic nervous system. This helps a person respond better to "fight and flight" situations during high stress.

- Yoga balances the central nervous system, which leads to enthusiasm and peace of mind, leading to better decisions in life.

- Because it balances all of the systems of the body, yoga leads to joyful longevity.

The Emotional/Mental Benefits of Yoga

- Yoga balances emotions, leading to equanimity in favorable or unfavorable circumstances. It leads to a positive way of thinking to help boost creativity and mental focus.

- Yoga reduces stress and brings peace.

- Yoga promotes overall well-being

- Yoga offers relaxation and peace of mind.

The Spiritual Benefits of Yoga

- Yoga brings happiness and personal contentment by being "one" with the universe.

- Yoga promotes love for oneself and for others.

- Yoga brings wisdom to help distinguish between real and unreal projections of the cosmos.

Yoga is for all, irrespective of religion, nationality or gender.

Why is yoga gaining popularity?

Like many other forms of alternative therapy, the purpose of yoga is to help restore the body's sense of balance known in medical terms as "homeostasis". Homeostasis is a state in which the body is healthy in the physical and mental state and is able to readily respond to demands, whether inner or outer.

It's more than a mere physical thing. The body, mind, and spirit must be in harmony. This is something that traditional medicine did not historically address but is now beginning to use in conjunction with conventional treatments. A growing amount of research shows a strong link between yoga and successfully preventing and treating a number of chronic and common medical conditions. (see www.svyasa.org, www.divyayoga.com)

To understand further the depth of this science, a different perspective is needed. In the Vedic literature, the human body is explained to exist in the five different planes of consciousness explained in the diagram shown at right.

Who am I?

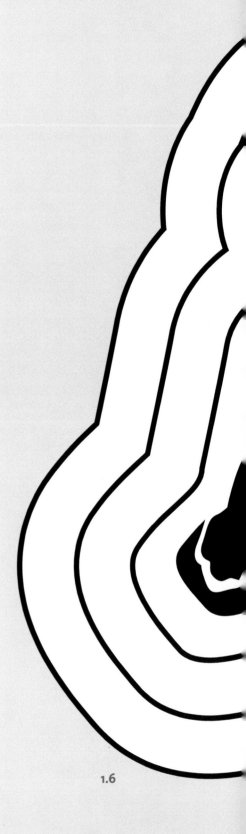

1.6

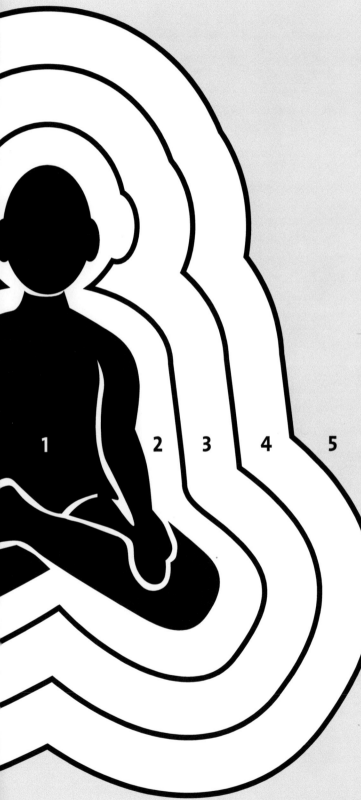

Concept of body

Map of Cosmic Consciousness
Who Am I?

Five Layers of Existence (Pança Kosha):

1. Annamaya Kosha: Physical sheath (body)

2. Pranamaya Kosha: Vital sheath (Body)

3. Manomaya Kosha: Astral sheath (body)

4. Vignanmaya Kosha: Wisdom sheath (body)

5. Anandmaya Kosha: Bliss sheath (Body)

Adapted from *Integrated Approach of Yoga Therapy for Positive Health*, by Dr. R Nagarathna & Dr. H. R. Nagendra, 2008.

"One should know oneself with one's own eye of wisdom. The self is within the five sheaths. The self has to be inquired into and eventually discarding the five sheaths by systematic, constant, and deep spiritual practices, self is realized.

~ Ramana Maharsi

"Pança Kosha"

One exists at different levels of consciousness or consciousness manifests itself at different levels of existence.

"Pança Kosha" or five levels of existence help us understand our presence from gross reality to the finest reality. It helps us understand the intricate inner world and the complex drama of life. What is seen and perceived by the gross senses seems so superfluous when the life and consciousness as a whole are understood.

Understanding of "Pança Kosha" also helps tremendously in meditation. When the meditator advances in his or her practices, the outer and grosser levels drop off from the feelings and true and unexplainable joy of self begins to be revealed. The meditator gets submerged in an ocean of pure nectar of existence: knowledge and love. The five layers of existence are explained as follows:

> *"Pança Kosha" or five levels of existence help us understand our presence from gross reality to the finest reality.*

1. Annamaya Kosha

This is the outermost or the most visible layer of existence, the body and its anatomy which you see. It is made up from the food (anna). It is the grossest of the existence.

2. Pranamaya Kosha

"Prana" means "bio or vital energy". Life is dependent on this layer. This layer gives body its functioning, physiology and vital force. This force or bio-energy is divided into the five major categories and five minor categories for its functioning. By doing Pranayama one can balance physiology and grow in life force.

Five major pranas – their location and functions:

(1) Prana: Above the umbilicus, around the heart (leads to enthusiasm, love, positive thinking)

(2) Apana: Below the umbilicus (perineum--anus) downward movement (responsible for excretion, negative thoughts)

(3) Vyana: Throughout the body (72,000 nadies or filaments of nervous system), Main Nadi is Sushumna in the middle of vertebrae, Ida on its left and Pingala on its right., Ida and Pingala are intertwined with each other.

(4) Udana: Around the heart, throat, palate, brain and in between. It is the upward movement of energy--last to leave at death

(5) Samana: At naval and surrounding area, balancing Prana and apana (digestion– balancing of thoughts)

Five minor pranas – up Pranas

(1) Kurma: controls eyelids and size of iris

(2) Krkala: controls sneezing and cough reflexes

(3) Devdatta: controls yawning

(4) Dhananjaya: produces phlegm

(5) Naga: relieves pressure on abdomen by belching, hiccups

3. Manomaya Kosha

The mind or the king of five senses makes this layer of existence. It is the mind which is the most powerful tool to help one understand the inner world. It is the mastery over this layer that one forgets the outer or gross world and dives into the deeper world of existence. The mind plays lots of tricks and it is very hard to control like a mad monkey, always busy thinking voluntarily and/or involuntarily thoughts, whether desirable or undesirable. So with incessant practice, understanding and discrimination, one learns to control the mind and then only one can enter into the deeper layers of existence.

4. Buddhimaya Kosha

Intelligence is the true property of every individual. It is shaped from the experiences of previous births and present experiences. From discrimination, good associations, and blessings from the great souls, it gets purified. It guides life and its direction.

5. Anandmaya Kosha

This is the innermost core of the human being, true joy, love and bliss. Irrespective of material presence, one is completely engrossed in the feeling of total fulfillment and inexpressible peace and happiness.

I am still beyond all these sheaths and I am the "self"

"This self cannot be cut, nor burnt, nor wetted, nor dried up. It is eternal, all pervading, stable, immovable and ancient."

Bhagwat Geeta - 2.24

Chapter 2: Yoga and the Preconception Stage

The decision to become a parent must be shared. With a thankful attitude, you and your spouse must pray together for a great soul to come to you as a child. Although it may seem difficult at first due to work and personal demands, as a couple, you must make the following lifestyle modifications to conceive your miracle child:

- Follow a yogic diet. This includes eating plenty of leafy green vegetables, lentils, and juices and whole grains in moderation, not drinking alcohol, and avoiding caffeine.

- Eat together if possible and early in the evening, preferably a few hours before going to sleep.

- Do not smoke or be around people who smoke.

- Do yoga together, preferably outdoors, daily for a minimum of 15 to 20 minutes, preferably 30 to 40 minutes.

- Walk together preferably outdoors at least three days a week for 35 to 40 minutes.

- Meditate every day ideally for 10 to 15 minutes, if not at least 5 minutes.

- Remember to pray together every day for the gift of a miracle child to come to you.

In the beginning you may feel that these lifestyle changes require a tremendous amount of willpower. After a short time, however, you'll see that yoga's unique ability to help you and your loved one, balance family/personal time and work time is well worth the effort. You'll also find that you're more relaxed, happy, and centered, the best way to conceive your miracle child. When you and your spouse are in a deep, loving relationship, you'll achieve true togetherness, of the mind, spirit, and body. You'll also share a prayerful attitude for the unborn soul to come.

In your own small way, *you and your spouse will play a vital role in creating a better future generation.*

Imagine A Mother

Imagine a mother who believes she belongs in the world.
A mother who celebrates her own life.
Who is glad to be alive.

Imagine a mother who celebrates the birth of her daughters.
A mother who believes in the goodness of her daughters.
Who nurtures their wisdom. Who cultivates their power.

Imagine a mother who celebrates the birth of her sons.
A mother who believes in the goodness of her sons.
Who nurtures their kindness. Who honors their tears.

Imagine a mother who turns toward herself with interest.
A mother who acknowledges her own feelings and thoughts.
Whose capacity to be available to her family deepens as she is available to herself.

Imagine a mother who is aware of her own needs and desires.
A mother who meets them with tenderness and grace.
Who enlists the support of respectful friends and chosen family members.

Imagine a mother who lives in harmony with her heart.
A mother who trusts her impulses to expand and contract.
Who knows that everything changes in the fullness of time.

Imagine a mother who embodies her spirituality.
A mother who honors her body as the sacred temple of the spirit of life.
Who breathes deeply as a prayer of gratitude for life itself.

Imagine a mother who values the women in her life.
A mother who finds comfort in the company of women.
Who sets aside time to replenish her woman-spirit.

Imagine yourself as this mother.

~ Patricia Lynn Reilly

Imagine a Mother © Patricia Lynn Reilly, M. Div., 2000,
reprinted with the permission of the author.

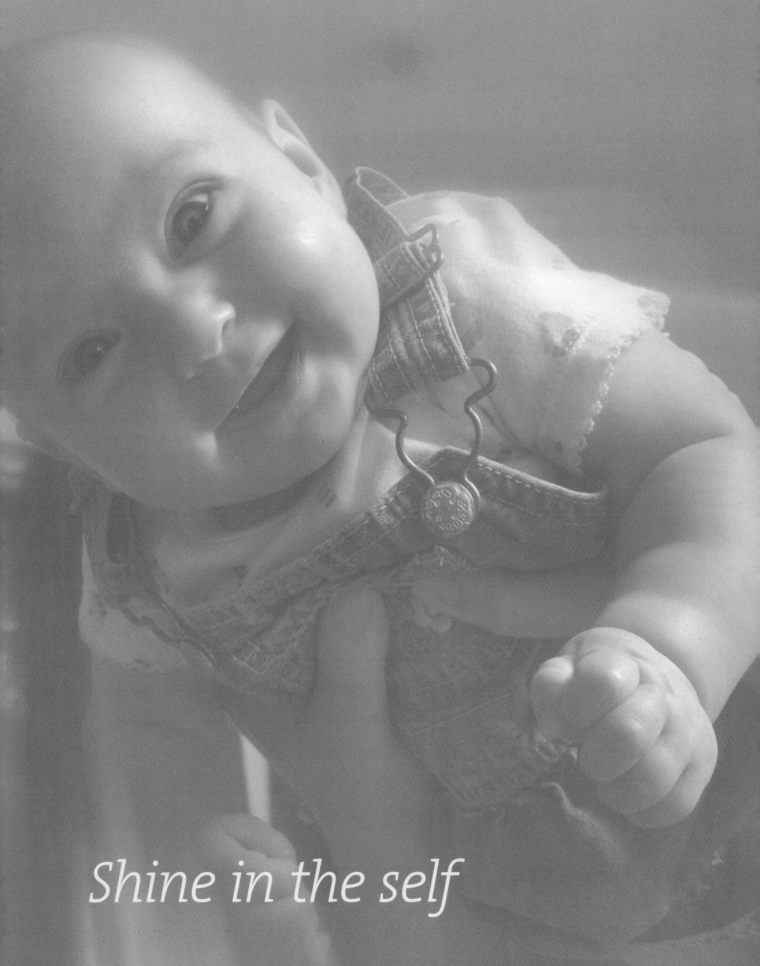

Shine in the self

Chapter 3: Yoga and Pregnancy

Pregnancy is the highest creative period of a woman's life. It's feminine energy, known as "prakriti," at its highest level manifested from absolute energy, known as "purusha."

A pregnant woman is given a wonderful gift, the gift of connecting with another soul that is looking for love and guidance. By feeling positive, confident, and harmonized, the expectant mother creates a rich, loving atmosphere in which the miracle child is nourished, physically, intellectually and emotionally. Unfortunately, modern obstetrics does not emphasize emotional nourishment.

Of all the methods available to help couples have a healthy pregnancy, an easy birth, a miracle child, and a healthy family unit, yoga has the most to offer. Words fall short to convey the value of yoga during pregnancy. This is because the science of yoga harmonizes the physiology of the voluntary/ involuntary muscles; the nervous system;

the urogenital system; the gastrointestinal system; the endocrine system; the respiratory system; the joints; and the circulatory systems to the mind and beyond. In other words, yoga is a multi-systems balancing multi-layer existence approach. It gives one understanding and acceptance of physiological changes, which cannot be achieved in any other way. This adds to true joy, confidence and enthusiasm.

After conception, a child will grow in his or her mother's womb for 280 days or 40 weeks. Every physiological and mental change in the mother will lead to corresponding changes in the growing fetus. From its inception, the fetus is deeply sensitive. The pregnant woman must nurture the new life inside her by doing yoga daily. All of the positive thoughts, creativity, and security gained from yoga will be channeled to the fetus. You will enjoy the synergy of mutually nourishing and exchanging energy by talking, feeling, and guiding the new life within.

Joy with pregnancy

3.1

A pregnant woman is given a wonderful gift, the gift of connecting with another soul that is looking for love and guidance.

You will learn to focus your mind and become aware of yourself as a new being, one in harmony with nature and the world. You will achieve great inner strength and faith so that you can face labor and motherhood without any fear.

By doing daily yoga and following a yogic lifestyle, you will embrace the changes pregnancy brings. You will learn to focus your mind and become aware of yourself as a new being, one in harmony with nature and the world. You will achieve great inner strength and faith so that you can face labor and motherhood without any fear.

Common symptoms of pregnancy, including morning sickness, fatigue, mood swings, constipation, anxiety, headache, stiffness, and pain, also are lessened or relieved through yoga. Your energy level will be boosted dramatically. Your body posture will become more balanced and relaxed. Yoga also helps improve flexibility of the joints and muscles, widens the pelvis and pelvic floor, and balances the gravitational center and vertebral pull.

Pregnancy enhances the self-development and spiritual evolution of a woman. Yoga helps quiet the mind to hone in on one's innermost feelings. You become more intuitive and focused. You feel empowered and wholesome. You learn to let go and surrender.

Fathers should be very knowledgeable and sensitive to the changes their spouses are going through. They should give full support and practice healthy lifestyle changes to make their pregnant wives feel loved and cherished. It's hard work carrying a baby, and husbands should be involved from the start to ease the process.

The baby's room should be prepared with soft colors in a quiet area with lots of circulating fresh air.

When choosing an obstetrician, it's imperative to pick one with a thinking process similar to yours. The entire process of wholesomeness should be brought out with minimal intervention. Labor and delivery should be conducted in a medical facility, like a hospital, where, if needed, measures for the surgery and neonatology care are available.

Overall the idea is to be in the most natural and friendly surroundings with minimal intervention, but at the same time, not ignoring modern medical help when necessary.

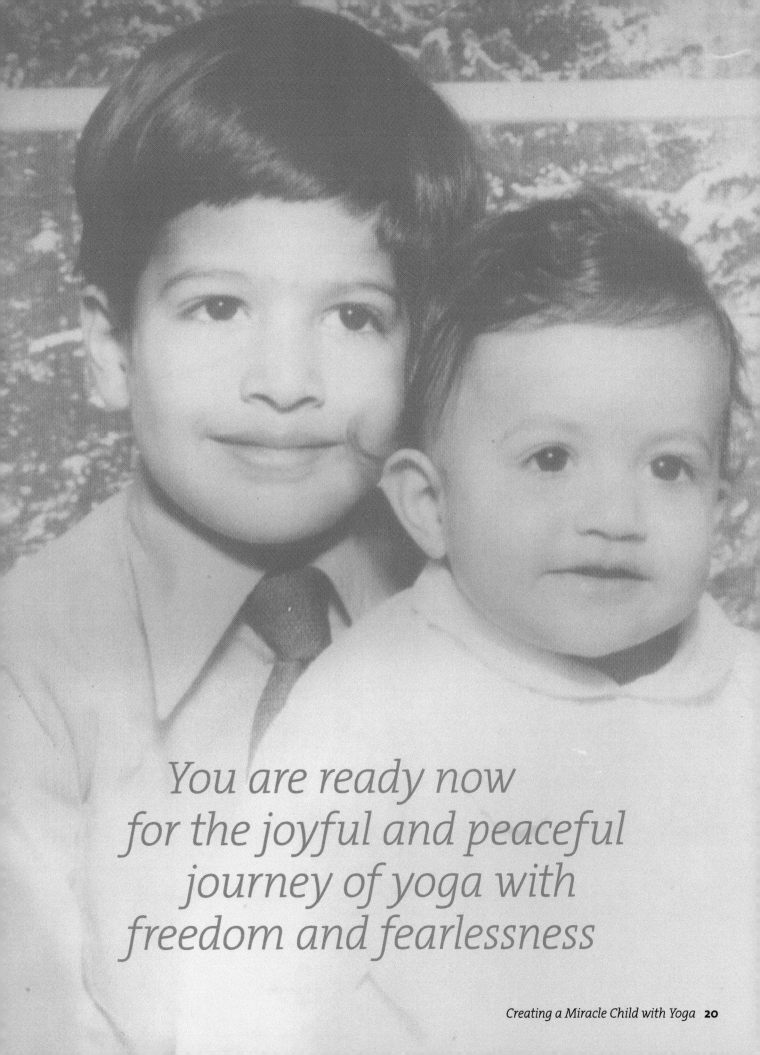

*You are ready now
for the joyful and peaceful
journey of yoga with
freedom and fearlessness*

Chapter 4: Yogic Postures for Pregnancy (Asanas)

"An asana is a steady and comfortable posture. By lessening the natural tendency for restlessness and by meditating on the infinite, posture is mastered."

~ Patanjali Yoga Sutras: 2:46-47

The ultimate aim of all asanas is to achieve physical fitness and the ability to sit for the long duration for the purpose of meditating to achieve tranquility of mind, which is necessary to achieve bliss and happiness. To gain the full benefit of asanas, aim for a full 45-minute yoga session daily. This daily session will include asanas, Pranayama, and short meditation. If this isn't possible, do two 20 minute sessions. You may also separate meditation time for 10 minutes or so before going to bed. Practice Pranayama in the beginning of each yoga session. Both you and your partner should do yoga to promote unity and personal growth.

An asana is a posture that enables you to sit firmly and comfortably, particularly for meditation. It is the systematic movement of the body. "Postures" help to penetrate the different layers of existence. With awareness it helps to reach consciousness. "Asanas" (postures) remove collected impurities from the muscles and joints and increase lisozymes in the brain, leading to feeling of freshness. Do you need to practice asanas? This is the question usually asked by some people. Of course, yogic asanas are very helpful to our body. To explain, here is a comparison of yogic asanas and other physical exercises:

Yogic Asanas:

1. Aim to achieve sense of well-being & homeostasis.
2. Usually static in nature (stretching).
3. Movements are slow, steady, and smooth.
4. It is done as per individual's capacity.
5. It requires minimum space.
6. Usually it does not require any equipment except a mat, few towels, and at times blocks for some people.
7. It cultivates spiritual advancement.
8. Yamas and Niyamas are prerequisites for yoga exercises (see details in Chapter 1).
9. Meditation and concentration are the ultimate aim of posture. This way it is a total lifestyle change.
10. Asanas are preparatory for higher yogic practices like meditation.
11. It is psycho-physiological in nature along with discipline.
12. Parasympathetic and sympathetic nervous system is balanced.
13. Energy expenditure is minimum but in the total yogic lifestyle, along with yogic diet, there is a total balance of body weight and body-mind and spirit.
14. It does not cause fatigue and injury.
15. It is not competitive, if at all, it is of a positive nature.
16. Possible to practice throughout life.
17. Non-stressful, optimum method of exercise.
18. Yoga refreshes.
19. Arteries and veins remain soft and elastic.
20. Cardiac nerves are rested and heart rate is steady.
21. There is no breathlessness.
22. Lungs become strong and are less affected by climate, altitude, and infections.
23. There is no depletion of hormones.
24. Kidney function is regulated due to direct organ massage and alteration in renal flow.
25. Improves digestion and assimilation of food.

Physical Exercise

1. Aim to achieve physical fitness.
2. Usually dynamic in nature.
3. Usually involves fast movements.
4. It is performed to others' standards.
5. Usually it requires large facility.
6. Usually it depends on modern equipment as in a gymnasium.
7. Spirituality is not involved.
8. Attitude adjustment not part of it.
9. It involves concentration.
10. Physical exercise may be undertaken to prepare for sports competition.
11. It emphasizes muscular training and discipline.
12. Sympathetic nervous system is stimulated.
13. It consumes lots of energy.
14. It may lead to fatigue and injury.
15. May have more of a spirit of competition.
16. At old age, possible to practice with limitations only.
17. Stress is possible.
18. Physical exercise may exhaust.
19. Arteries and veins may become hard.
20. Cardiac nerves are stimulated and heart rate is fast and changed.
21. There is breathlessness.
22. Effect of physical exercise on lungs is comparatively less.
23. There is depletion of hormones.
24. Intensive physical exercise does not regulate kidney function.
25. May not affect digestion.

Follow these principles during your yogic exercises:

- Wear loose clothing and no jewelry of any kind.

- Choose a quiet place, preferably in the open air uniting with nature. In winter, a quiet corner of any room will do. Try to keep the same place, if possible.

- Perform asanas on an empty stomach (at least two hours without eating). Drinking water or juice is okay - only if necessary.

- Practice asanas right after taking a bath (if possible) for easier body movement.

- Use a carpet or yoga mat.

- Calm the mind by doing 15 minutes of pranayama before asanas may help to do postures better - but it is an individual's preference.

- If you're tired, in a heavy mood, or under stress, do not do posture practice, except Shavasana.

- Always coordinate asanas with full, deep breathing.

- Focus on "being," aware of your mind and body.

- You may do loosening exercises before doing asanas.

- Do the asanas to the best of your capacity and slowly. (It doesn't matter how many asanas you perform at a given time. Respect your body. Do not overdo. But be consistent.)

- According to Patanjali, at the end of each asana you must establish yourself in a natural state without effort. Your aim is to elevate your mind to the spiritual field and to dwell in the principle of the infinite, which is yoga's goal.

- All asanas are not recommended for everyone. Some of them should be avoided by those with heart disease, high blood pressure, and certain other medical conditions.

- Practice and achieve deep relaxation at the end.

- Ground your energy into the earth by transferring some of your weight into the ground, just like a plant sending down roots.

- As a general principle whenever you do a bending down posture, you breathe out. While performing a posture that moves the body up, breathe in. If you bend to one side, you must bend to the other side to balance the muscles.

- The Pranayama session also can be performed by itself or before or after postures. It doesn't always have to be followed by asanas. Some people like to spend 20 to 30 minutes before going to bed doing Pranayama (anuloma/viloma) and meditation. If time does not permit, then try doing several short sessions over the course of a day. Remember to learn and mix different breathing techniques and postures.

It's also important to make other members of the family aware of your need to be healthy and happy through yoga. They also can be part of your yogic exercise team. But doing yoga alone also can be wonderful. You develop a relationship with your super-consciousness and can really enjoy the peace, love, confidence, and internal strength gained by that bond.

A.) Fine muscular and joint movement exercises (Loosening exercises)

The postures (asanas) are grouped for your understanding and are depicted by photos. You may like to mix and match the different asanas on different days as per your physical needs, desire, and availability of time. Try to start with or end with pranayama. This will help you to center yourself to "being" one with your awareness--consciousness.

Standing (Loosening)

1. **Standing with ease:** Due to the pregnant state, it's important to learn how to properly stand. With feet wide apart, with slow breath with awareness, stand with ease, release your vertebrae, and relax the muscles of both feet. Keep yourself well grounded to the floor, with your hands relaxed, and enjoy pulling energy from cosmos with breathing in and relax with breathing out.

A.) Fine muscular and joint movement exercises (Loosening exercises)

B.) Standing postures

C.) Sitting postures

D.) Lying postures

E.) Pelvic floor widening postures

F.) Relaxation--winding down

G.) Grounding

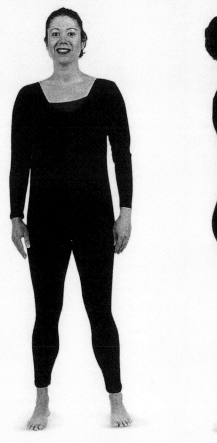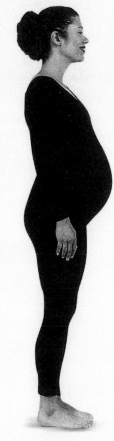

4.1   4.2

Practice becomes firmly grounded when well attended to for a long time, without break and in all earnestness.

~ *The Yoga Sutrast of Patanjali - 1.14*

Standing against the wall

2. Wall Standing: Gentle movement at the waist, bend forward and backward.

3. Hand stretch (forward): with fingers locked, going to the chest with breathing in and away from the chest with breathing out. (4.3 - 4.4)

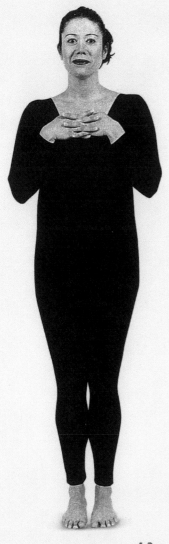

4.3

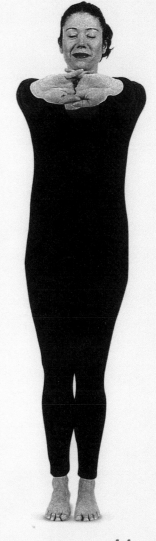

4.4

4. Hand stretch (45 degrees) same way.

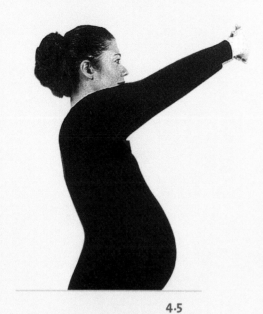

4.5

5. Hand stretch (90 degrees) same way.

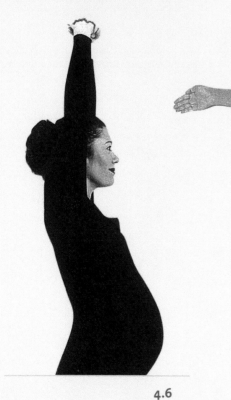

4.6

6. Hand stretch (in front): bring both palms together with breathing in and then separate them to 180 degrees with breathing out (do 10 times).

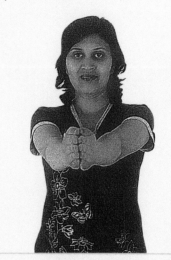

4.7

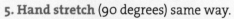

4.8

7. Ankle stretch breathing (go up on ankles and bring them down with breathing in and out (1st and early 2nd trimester only). In the 3rd trimester you may hold onto the chair for the support and with the legs spread hip width apart.

8. Toes and ankles: flexion and extension (alternate leg), also rotate the ankles clockwise and counterclockwise. Use the support of the chair or a countertop.

9. Fingers: (i) Flex and extend at finger joints (ii) full closing and opening of fists. (4.9 - 4.10)

10. Wrists: keep the elbows straight, with extended hands and closed fists, rotate wrists clockwise and counterclockwise.

11. Shoulder rolls: with fingers on the shoulders, rotate the elbows clockwise and counterclockwise with breathing. (4.11 - 4.12)

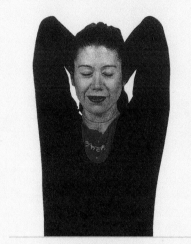

4.11

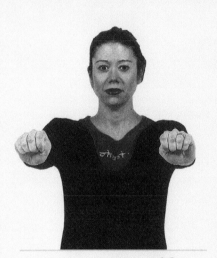

4.9

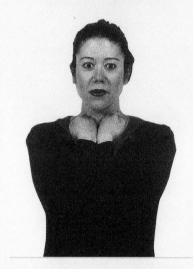

4.12

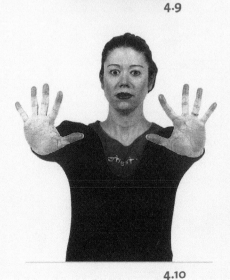

4.10

12. Neck rolls: rotate the neck slowly clockwise and counterclockwise with breathing in through half circle and breathing out through half circle.

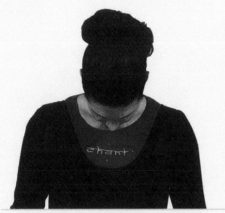

4.13

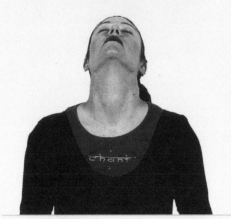

4.14

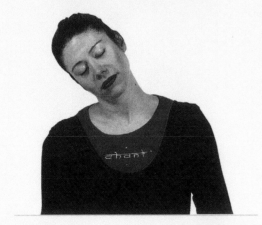

4.15

Sitting (Loosening)

1. Ankle flexion and extension and rotation clock and counterclockwise.

2. Basic sitting against wall.

3. Toes: flexion and extension.

4. Forward leaning, spread the legs. With extended hands breathe out, bend and touch the toes of the same side, alternatively later on touch the opposite toe with the legs wide apart, and then come up with breathing in. This loosens the lower back and hips. (1st and early 2nd trimester – later on modify)

5. Wrists, fingers, shoulders, and neck rolls. (Do same as in standing position)

6. Cradle the hip and move the hip joint from side to side.

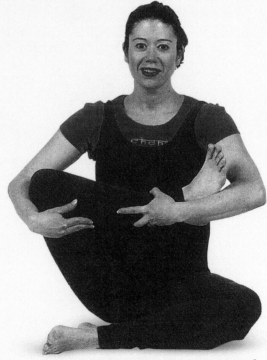

4.16

7. Then holding the foot with one hand and with the other hand bring the same side of the bent knee up and down. Repeat the same on the other side. This is great for the loosening of the hip joints.

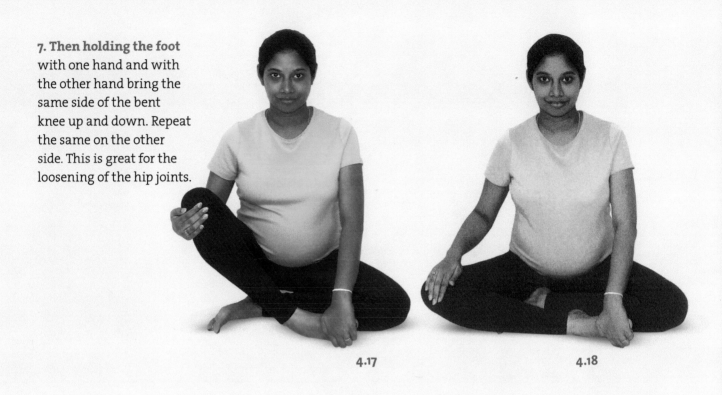

4.17   4.18

Lying   (Loosening)

Lying on the left lateral side, raise the leg 45 degrees. Do alternately on right side (only in 1st and early 2nd trimester). Strengthens lower abdominal and lower back muscles. Left lateral lying in later part of 2nd and 3rd trimester.

Raise both legs 45 degrees if possible in supine position. 1st trimester only.

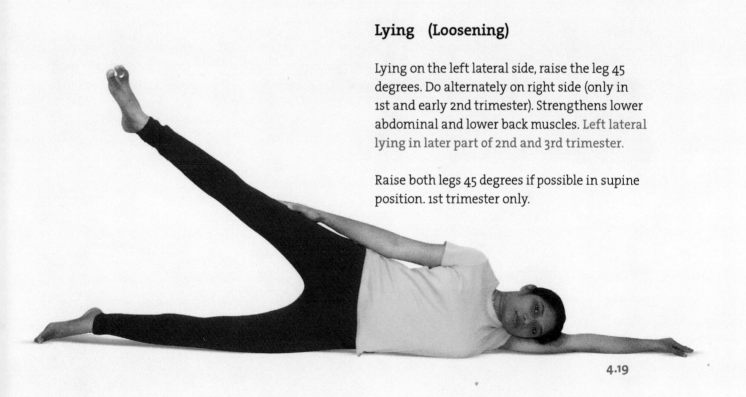

4.19

Postures (asanas)

B.) Standing poses

1. Balanced Standing pose (see loosening exercise)

2. Tree pose (Vrikshasana): see variations with the support of chair in the picture. It lengthens spines, increases concentration and intuitiveness, helps thigh and back muscles (4.21, 4.22, 4.23)

3. Side bending (Artha-kati Chakrasana): It helps flexibility of spine, improves lung, liver and spleen functions. It also increases linear awareness.

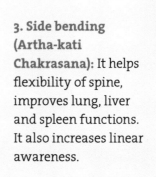

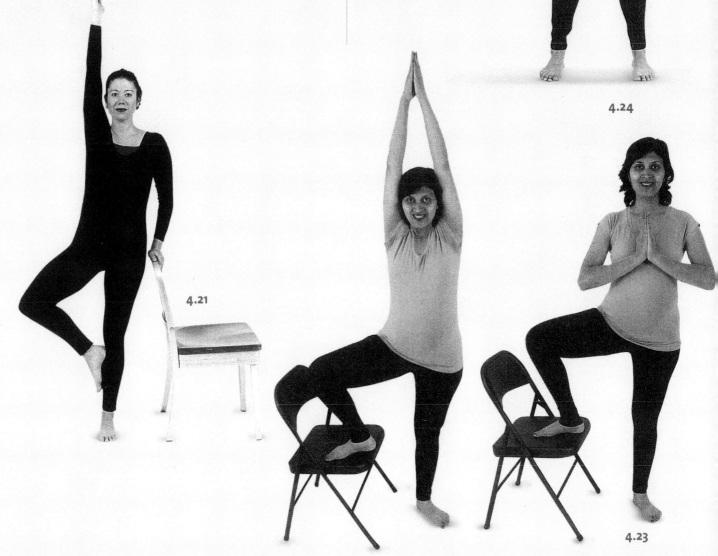

4.24

4.21

4.22

4.23

4. Triangular pose (Trikonasana): strengthens calf, thigh muscles and waist muscles, improves spine, removes back pain and vitalizes the kidneys.

- Ipsilateral: (same side) (4.26).
- Contralateral: (opposite side) Pari vrtta Trikonasana (4.25).
- Triangle forward bend in 3rd trimester. (with the support of chair) (4.28).

5. (Tadasana): stretches spine, improves intuitiveness, helps shoulder. Keep feet flat on the ground. In 1st and early 2nd trimester you may go up on your toes.

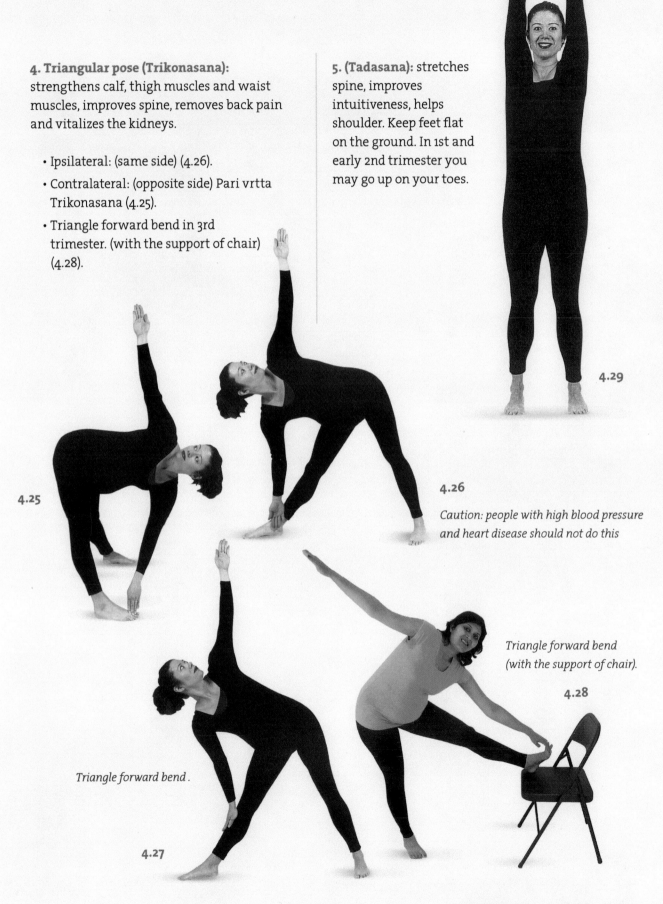

4.29

4.25

4.26

Caution: people with high blood pressure and heart disease should not do this

Triangle forward bend (with the support of chair).

4.28

Triangle forward bend .

4.27

7. Warrior poses
Great for widening the lower birth canal, making thighs, calves and shoulders strong.

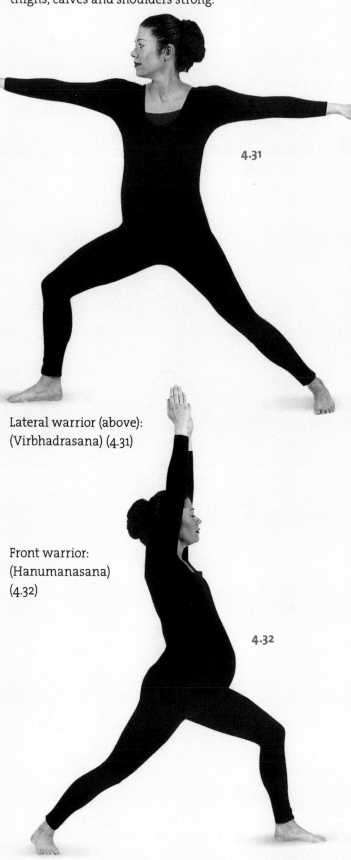

4.31

6. Knee strengthening (Sankatasana): It strengthens the knees and thighs. Spread the legs and go up and down by bending the knees with breathing in and out, keeping the torso straight up (in the 1st and early 2nd trimester you may like to go up and down on the toes) (4.30).

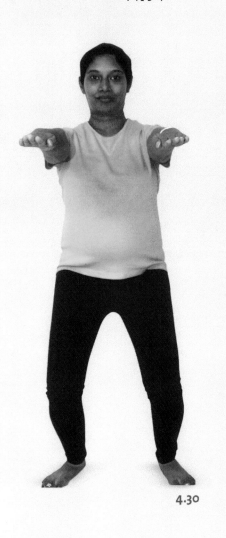

Lateral warrior (above): (Virbhadrasana) (4.31)

Front warrior: (Hanumanasana) (4.32)

4.32

4.30

8. Standing twist. Strengthening of back muscles and spine

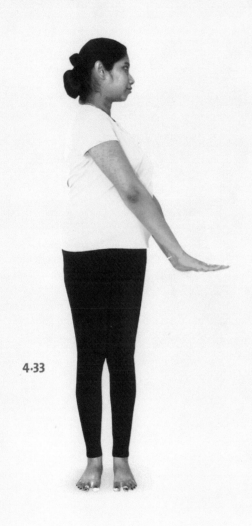

4.33

9. Forward bend: (Pad Hastasana) with or without knee bend, makes the spine flexible, strengthens the thigh, and prevents constipation.

Caution: People with high blood pressure and heart diseases should not do this. People with any spine problems or herniated disc should also avoid forward bending.

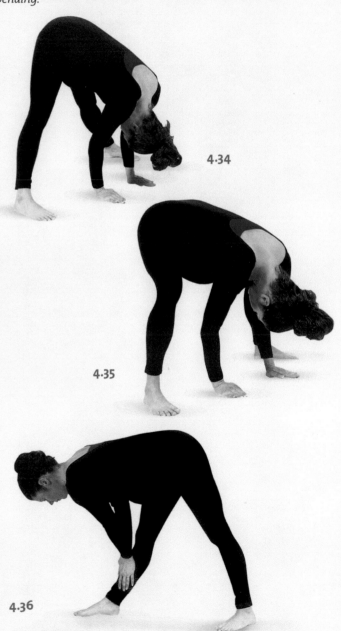

4.34

4.35

4.36

10. Moon pose (Backward bend): (Artha chakrasana): helps to expand the chest and cures neck and upper back pain, improves intestinal functions, promotes circulation of blood into head.

11. Yoga Mudra (Standing): great for the shoulders and lower back (in 1st and early 2nd trimester).

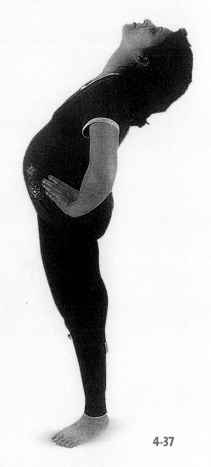

4.37

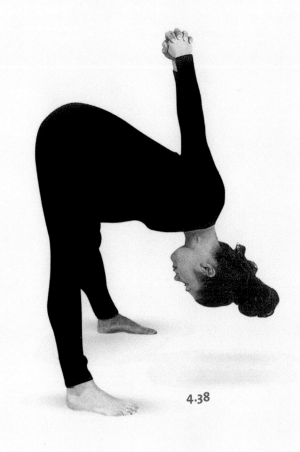

4.38

Caution: People with vertigo should avoid this pose.

Caution: people with high blood pressure, heart disease, and people with spinal problems should avoid this.

12. Standing Squat: Great for thighs, lower back and pelvic widening.

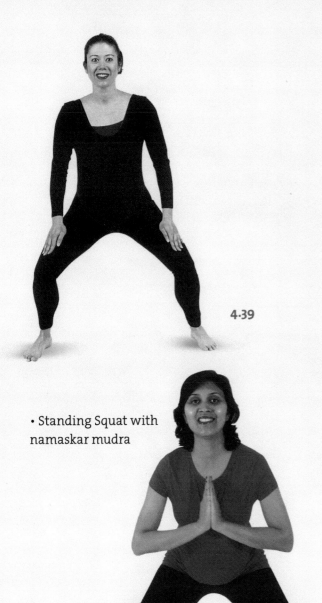

4.39

• Standing Squat with namaskar mudra

4.40

"Yoga is not the physical exercises; it is changing lifestyle, changing mental attitude to positive way and, ultimately penetrating deep into the consciousness."

c.) Sitting poses

1. Half angle pose: (Janu Sirsasana): massages abdominal organs, increases elasticity of spine, especially the lumbar, relieves sciatica, strengthens hamstrings by stretching, improves concentration and prana.

• half angle pose

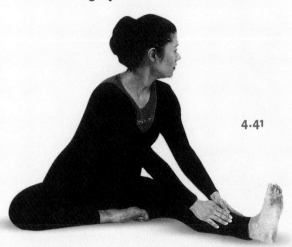

4.41

• modified half angle pose with arm in the back

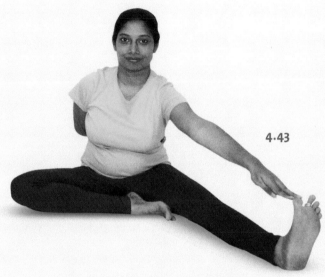

4.43

• half angle pose with yoga belt.

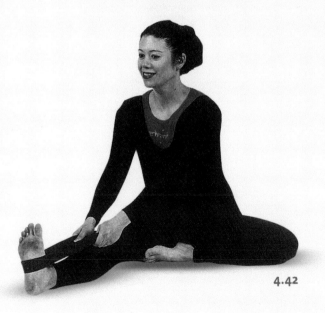

4.42

• modified half angle pose with one arm raised

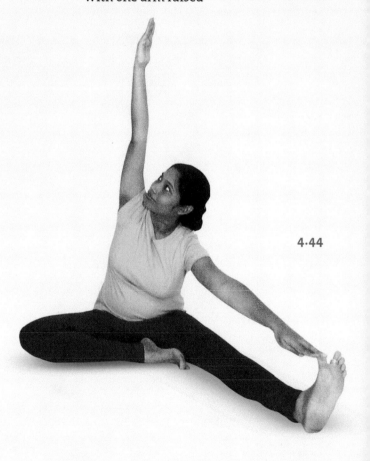

4.44

2. Lotus pose (Padmasana)

- Helps spine, back, improves concentration and intuitiveness.
- Half lotus: improves concentration, helps the spine and back. (4.45)
- Full lotus position (4.46)
- Twist in half lotus. (front view - 4.47)

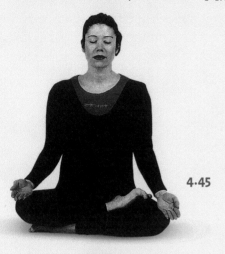

4.45

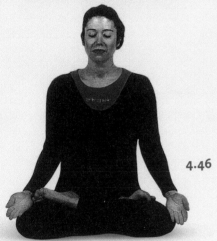

4.46

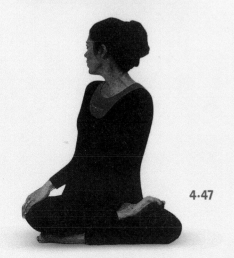

4.47

3. Cow pose: (Gau-mukhasana): strengthens shoulders, upper back, and upper arm muscles, controls urinary bladder and helps incontinence.

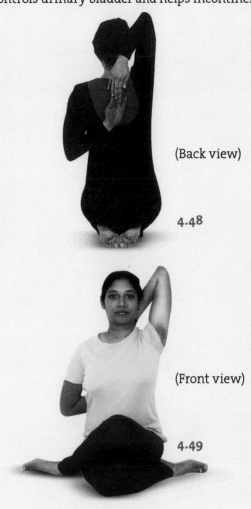

(Back view)

4.48

(Front view)

4.49

- One may use yoga belt as shown in the picture

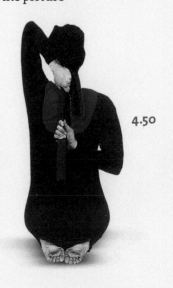

4.50

4. Tailor Sitting (Bhadrasana, Baddha Konasana): Helps widening of pelvis. Helps widening of introitus and strengthening of perineal and gluteal muscles and hip joints.

- Tailor sitting with a partner's feet in the back.
- Back to back with a partner.

5. Sitting with legs wide. (Upavishtha konasana)

- Forward bending. (see in pelvic widening poses - 4.75 and 4.76)
- Side bending, with different hand positioning: lengthens spine and chest, strengthens chest, back and neck muscles.
- Both hands holding toes (4.53).

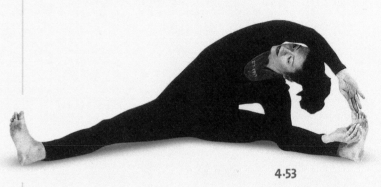

4.53

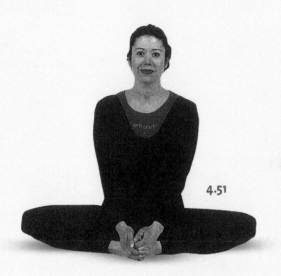

4.51

- One hand in front of other, raised to ceiling to lengthen the spine.
- One hand in front and other on the waist. (4.54)

- Movement with Bhadrasana (Butterfly): helps to widen the introitus and strengthen hip joints

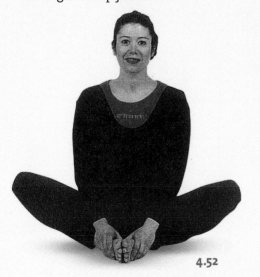

4.52

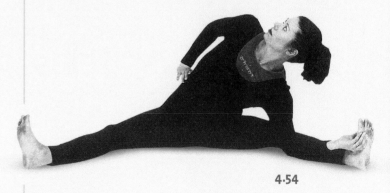

4.54

6. Kneeling: (Vajrasana): sitting on the heels with knees folded brings steadiness to the body. Good pose for meditation. It's the only pose that can be done even after eating. These poses lengthen and strengthen the spine as well as improve intuitiveness and concentration and improves digestion and prevents constipation.

- Basic kneeling: knees together (first and early 2nd trimester).
- Basic kneeling: knees wide apart (4.55) helps to relax in the sitting position.
- Basic kneeling: using bolster (4.56).
- Leaning forward: on to your elbows (first and early 2nd trimester). (see relaxation pose 4.84)
- Hands stretched forward: (Shashankasana) fully extended on the floor (first and early 2nd trimester). (see relaxation pose 4.83)
- Kneeling twist position: hands by the side of the body (4.57).
- Basic kneeling with hands in garudasana position (4.58).
- Basic kneeling with hands in "Namaskar mudra" (4.59).

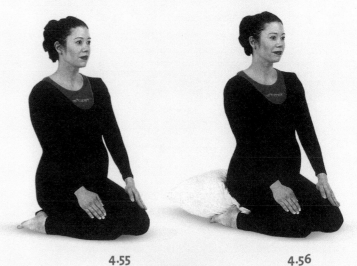

4.55   4.56

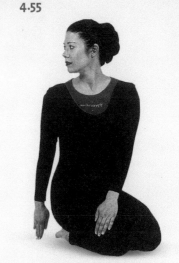

4.57

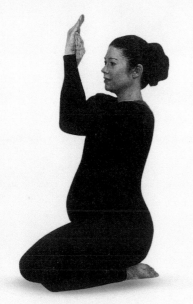

4.58

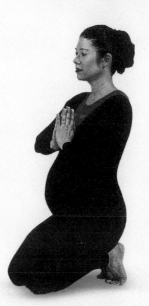

4.59

7. Squatting (Malasana): squatting poses are very important. Squatting helps perineal muscles get stronger, widens introitus or vaginal opening. Upper thigh muscles get great exercise along with gluteal muscles it helps vertebre and neck muscles.

- (Sitting with palm in prayer position or clasped) (4.60)
- Sitting on a stool. (see pelvic widening 4.74)
- Squatting with support under the heels: helps pelvic floor muscles, as well as the vertebrae and neck muscles (4.61).
- Squatting on floor with holding onto a chair (4.62).
- Squatting with holding partner's hands (4.63).

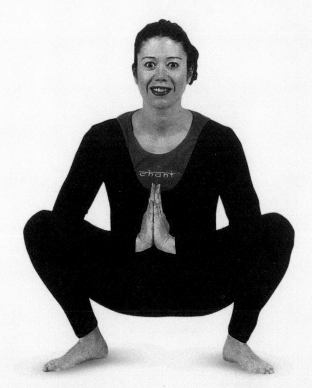

4.60

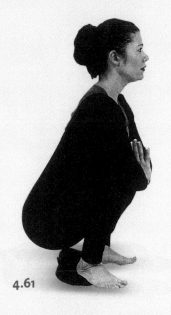

4.61

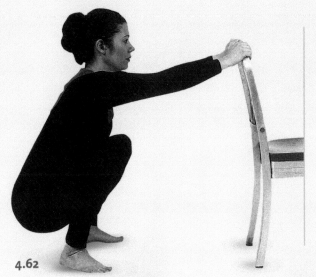

4.62

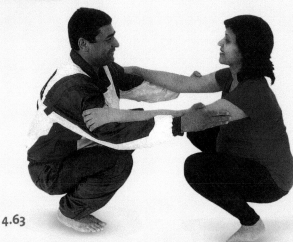

4.63

8. Garudasana: (arms only) in sitting or standing position: for shoulder strengthening and neck release.

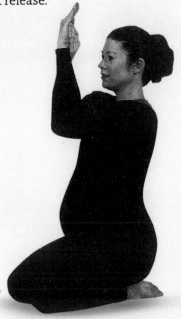

4.64

9. Spinal twist: great for the spine, upper back muscles, upper abdominal muscles and neck. Back hand supports the weight of the upper part of the body.

10. Camel pose: (modified Ustrasana): with the help of chair, spread the knees, hold onto the chair. Great for the neck, upper and middle back and spines. (Do gently. Hold 20-30 seconds, 2-5 times).

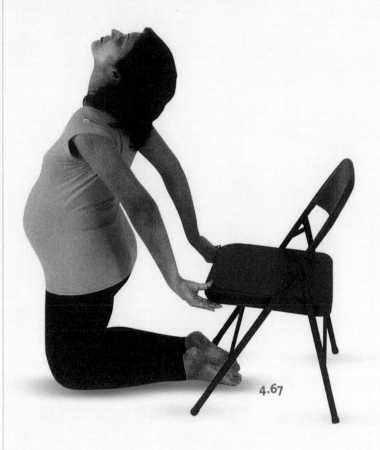

4.67

(Front view)
4.65

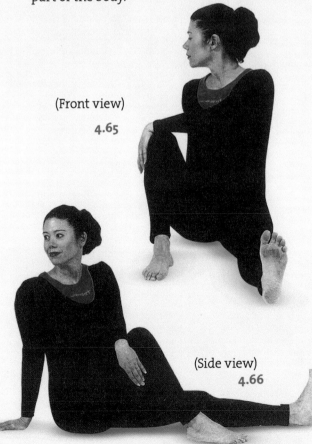

(Side view)
4.66

D.) Lying poses

General Principle: supine position only in 1st trimester and left lateral position in late 2nd and 3rd trimester to help the circulation in the mother and the fetus.

1. Shoulder stand (Sarvangasana): with support of the wall. (1st and early 2nd trimester, later on with caution) (4.68)

Caution: If you start to feel dizzy - release the pose and turn to the left side.

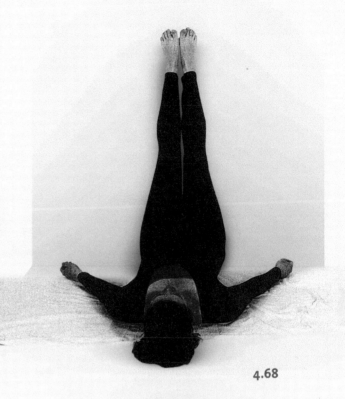

4.68

• Modified Sarvangasana: half leaning against the wall with knees bent. (1st and early 2nd trimester, later on with caution) (4.69)

Caution: If you start to feel dizzy - release the pose and turn to the left side.

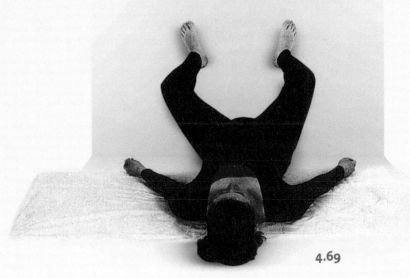

4.69

Widening in lying position, while enjoying the gravity in lying on the back with body comfortable - widening of legs with support helps birth canal to open more. It also helps varicose veins of legs.

4. Modified Boat pose (Naukasana) with support of elbows: strengthens the lower back and abdominal muscles, stabilizes umbilicus.

4.72

2. Lower half back raise (Setubandhanasana): great for the strengthening of back muscles and for lower backache.

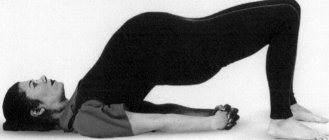

4.70

5. Shavasana (in left lateral position) for the total relaxation.

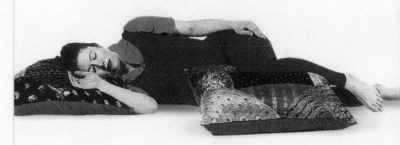

4.73

3. Neck extension in lying (peacock position) with support of elbows: this pose is difficult in the later part of pregnancy, but helps a great deal in lessening neck and upper back pain.

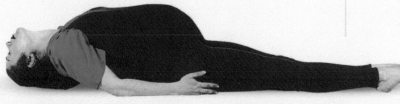

4.71

E.) Pelvic floor widening poses

1. Squatting (Malasana): Squatting poses are very important because they help perineal muscles to get stronger; they widen introitus or vaginal opening. Upper thigh muscles get great exercise along with gluteal muscles.

- Squatting in standing: (see standing poses (4.39 - 4.40)
- Squatting in sitting: with variations. (see sitting poses (4.60 & 4.61 & 4.62 & 4.63)
- Squatting on stool (4.74)

2. Warrior poses: (Virabhadrasana and Hanumanasana)

These poses are great for widening of lower birth canal, making thighs strong. (see standing poses 4.31 & 4.32)

3. Tailor sitting: (Baddha Konasana or Bhadrasana): (see sitting poses. 4.51 & 4.52)

These help again widening of introitus and strengthening of hip joints. It is helpful and joyful to do this with the partner.

4. Sitting against the wall with legs widely stretched: (Upavishtha Konasana) (4.75 & 4.76)

Simple sitting with legs wide apart helps widening of pelvis with total relaxation.

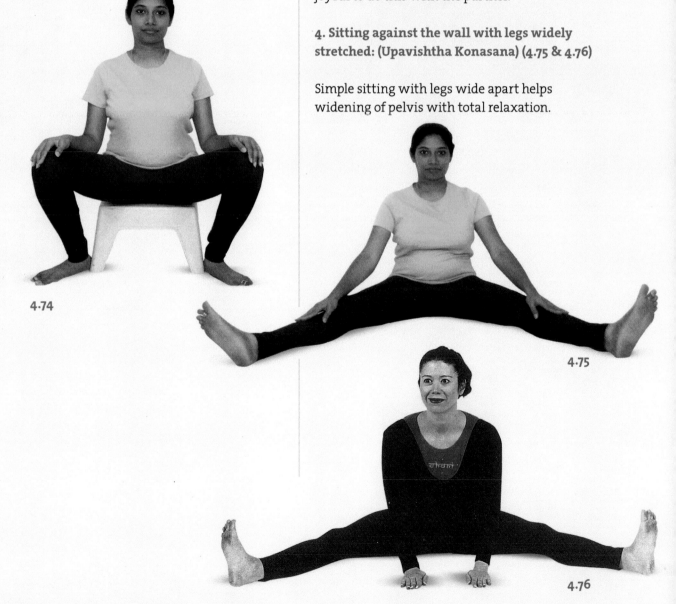

4.74

4.75

4.76

"The practice of asanas purges the body of its impurities, bringing strength, firmness, calm, and clarity of mind."

~ *B.K. S. Ayengar*

7. Standing with legs and hands apart.

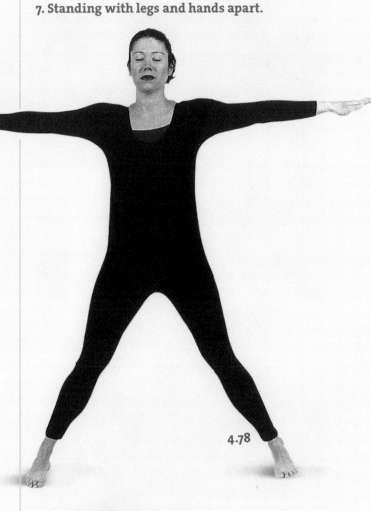

4.78

5. Widening in lying position: (Modified Sarvangasna) (see lying poses. 4.68 & 4.69)

While enjoying the gravity in lying on the back with body comfortable, widening of legs with support helps birth canal to open more. It also helps varicose veins of legs. Lying on the back with legs wide apart with knees bent and half leaning against the wall.

(These can be done in 1st and early 2nd trimester)

6. Lying with legs in the frog position.

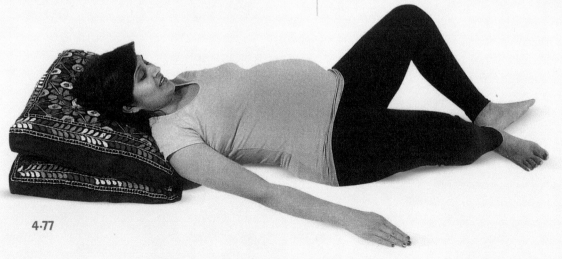

4.77

F.) Relaxation poses

1. Lying on left side: with pillow. In the later part of pregnancy, always be on the left side of the body to help blood return to the heart from the lower part of the body (4.79).

- Lying with beanbag (4.80).
- Sitting with beanbag.
- Lying with legs in frog position (see pelvic widening - 4.77)

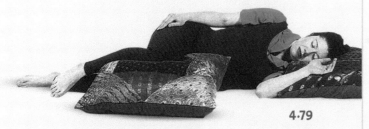

4.79

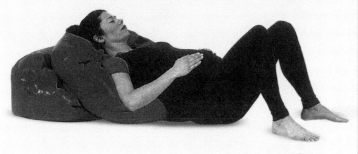

4.80

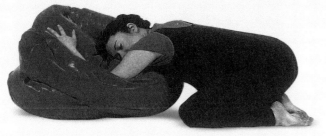

4.81

2. Sitting relaxation pose

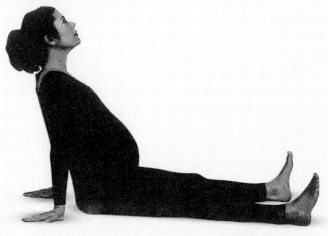

4.82

3. Basic kneeling with hands stretched forward: Shashankasana. (1st & 2nd trimester, modify for the 3rd trimester on bean bag)

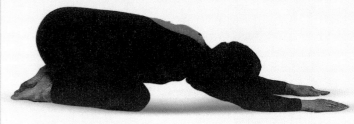

4.83

4. Basic kneeling leaning forward on elbows

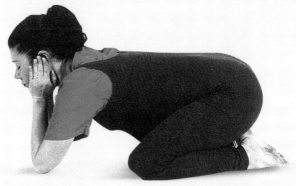

4.84

G.) Grounding

It is important to practice what to do after the relaxation stage of yoga. This is called grounding. Roll over on the lateral side of the body and slowly come up.

Ground yourself before getting up. Always use a simple ritual to mark the transition between your yoga session and the next item on your agenda. You may recite a small ending prayer or "mantra". Grounding can also be as simple as rubbing both the palms hard together and then cupping the warm palms over your eyes. Taking stock of how you feel after your yoga session is completed is also grounding. Grounding also is tidying up your yoga space.

What's important is to make this transition. If you don't, you may lose the peacefulness achieved through yoga. The deeper your relaxation, the more important it is to come out of it slowly and completely before moving on to something else.

*Postpartum yogic asanas
(see chapter 10)*

Yoga balances all the physiological systems of the body, leading to joyful longevity.

Chapter 5: Yogic Breathing Techniques (Pranayama)

"That firm posture being acquired, the movements of inhalation and exhalation should be controlled. This is pranayama."

~ *Patanjali Yoga Sutras: 2:49*

Breath is a bridge between the mind and body.

That's why it's so important to learn the following breathing techniques called "Pranayama." Pranayama practices expand and control the flow of "prana," which means life force. Prana helps to balance the total physiology of the body.

You should learn all of the following Pranayama for pregnancy and incorporate them into your daily yoga routine. "Prana" is the energy. "Ayama" is directing and expanding of this energy. Regular and correct practice with mindfulness brings true success and joy. Always try to do pranayama with a totally relaxed attitude. Sit on the floor or on a chair, in a quiet place, sit tall for the upward flow of the energy in your spine. This will lead to true bliss. A proper and regular practice of Pranayama also brings blood pressure down, lowers anxiety, improves digestion, and increases mental peace. Overall oxygenation of all the cells of the body improves with the improvement of the proper cell function and increase in energy.

"Prāṇsyedam Vaśe sarvam tridivid pratishitam, Māteva putrān raksasva śrīśca prajnam ca vidhehi na Iti"

It means "Whatever is there in the universe, within or beyond our cognition, is all in the control of Prana. Oh Prana! Protect us as a mother protects her child with affection. Provide us wealth and wisdom."

~ *Prasnopanisad 2/13*

1. Deep Breathing

The goal of deep breathing is to breath with awareness, ease, and expand the chest. It should be performed in a sitting position with or without back support. Keep your back, neck, and head straight to better channel the energy flow from the bottom of the spine upward to the head. Start by closing your eyes and focusing your mental eye on the tip of your nose or between your eyebrows. Breathe in slowly and fully from the nose to chest to abdomen and then breathe out fully by pulling your abdomen in and then through the chest and through the nose. Ideally the time to exhale should be twice the time to inhale. Repeat the slow, smooth, continuous breathing several times. 15 to 20 times. Takes 1 to 2 minutes. See diagram below.

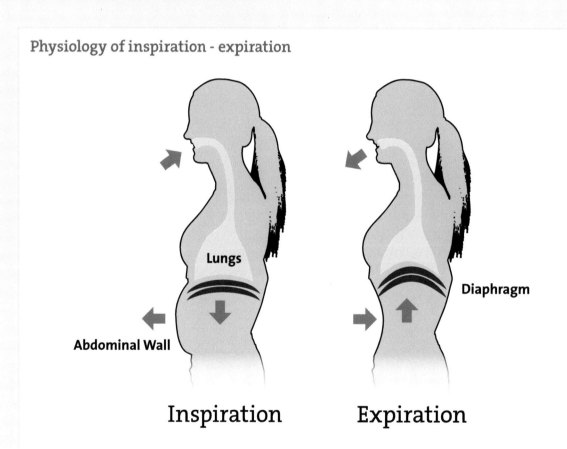

Physiology of inspiration - expiration

Lungs

Diaphragm

Abdominal Wall

Inspiration   Expiration

- With breathing in lungs expand, the diaphragm moves down, the abdominal visceras are pushed down and abdominal wall comes out.

- With breathing out the lungs get compressed due to the rising of the diaphragm, abdominal visceras get more space, and abdominal wall gets pulled in.

5.1

2. Anuloma-Viloma (Alternate Nostril Breathing)

The goal of Anuloma-Viloma breathing is to balance the right and left nostrils, and through them, the balance of two sides of the brain. The right side of the brain is intuitive, with love, emotion, creativity and compassion. The left side of the brain is related to logic, intellect, enthusiasm, courage and organizational skills. Metabolically right is the "Solar" nostril with catabolic activities and left is the "Lunar" nostril with anabolic activities. With this pranayama solar and lunar energies are balanced. It should be performed in a sitting position either on the floor or on a chair.

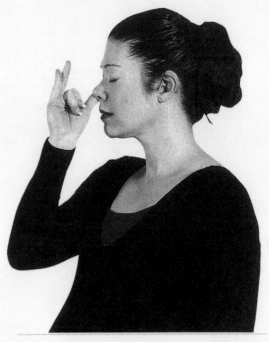

5.2

Start by closing the right nostril with your right thumb. Breathe in deeply, slowly, and fully through the left nostril, then close the left nostril with your middle and ring fingers and breathe out fully and slowly through the right nostril. Then breathe in through the right nostril and then close the right nostril again with the right thumb, breathing fully out through the left nostril. This is one round of "Anuloma-Viloma." Repeat the sequence for 5 to 10 minutes.

The important thing to remember is you always start breathing in through the left nostril and end the practice by breathing out through the left nostril. Another important point to remember is, whichever nostril you breathe out, subsequently breathe in with the same nostril.

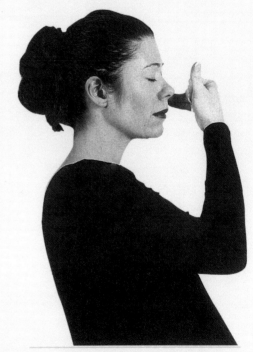

5.3

3. Three Stage Breathing

Three stage breathing is practiced to expand all the lobes of the lungs to achieve full-capacity breathing. This is especially important during labor to help ease labor pains.

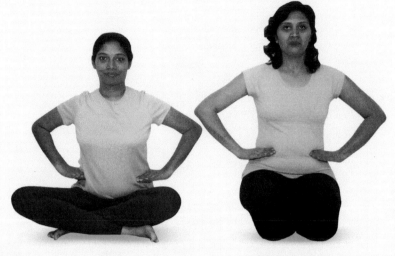

5.4

Lower lobe or abdominal breathing helps to expand the lower lobes of the lungs. Start by keeping your hands at your waist with your fingers in front and your thumbs in back. Breathe in fully and notice that the tips of your fingers move apart when you breathe in. When you exhale, notice how the tips of your fingers move together. Repeat the sequence 10 times.

Chest breathing should be practiced the same way: Keep your thumbs under your armpits and fingers horizontally in the front of your chest. Broaden your chest by breathing in slowly, deeply, and continuously, then breathe out. Note the separation of fingers with breathing in. Repeat the sequence 10 times.

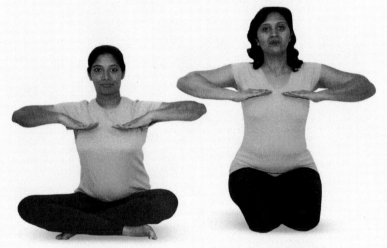

5.5

Clavicular or Upper Lobe breathing: Repeat the previous sequence with your hands on your upper back with your elbows folded and pointing to the ceiling, both little fingers and the palms touching each other. Breathe in and out deeply and slowly. Repeat the sequence 10 times.

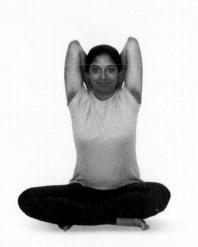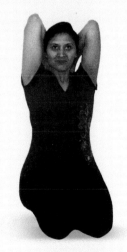

5.6

4. Cat Stretch Breathing

Make a table top – on two hands and two knees separated hip width approximately 18" to 24" apart. Breathe in. Turn head up and a little forward by extending the neck up and bring the middle of the back down. Hold the breath to the count of 10. Then breathe out and bring the chin to the chest and push the back up and a little back like an angry pushy cat. (Repeat 10 times) This breathing is great for strengthening of the back and for back pain. (Do 5-10 times)

You may lift up the leg with breathing in and bring the leg down with breathing out. You may also hold the leg as shown in the picture. (5.9 & 5.10)

5. Bhramari breathing
(Humming Bee Pranayama):

Bhramari breathing helps achieve intuitiveness and unity with the source, unity of the mind, and unity with consciousness. It creates a stress-free mind, one with peace and harmony. Sit in an erect (firm but not tense) position with your back, neck, and head in one line. Keep the index finger of both hands above your eyebrows, and reamining of three fingers cupped gently on your eyes. The thumb closes the external ear only during exhalation. Breathe in deep, then close the ears, and breathe out long and smooth with a humming bee sound. (Takes 1 to 2 minutes, do 5-10 times).

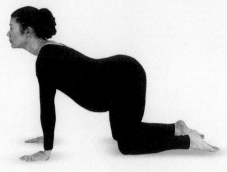

5.7

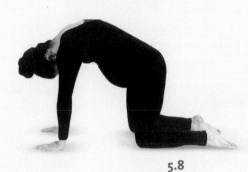

5.8

5.9

5.10

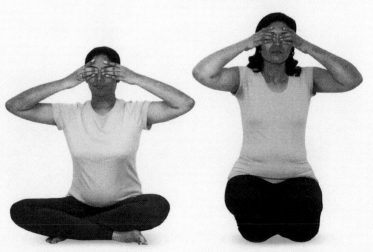

5.11

6. Primodial Sound (AUM) Pranayama

Breathe in deep and then breathe out long with the sound "AUM" starting from the depth of abdomen to the chest through the mouth, by ending with the sound of "MA" by closing your lips. This takes you to the deeper layers of unity and potentiates your peacefulness. (Takes 1 to 2 minutes – do 5 to 10 times)

7. Left Nostril Breathing: Optional

Left nostril breathing creates a balance of emotion, love, compassion, and forgiveness. It is also anabolic. Start by breathing in slowly and deeply through the left nostril and breathe out through the same nostril. Repeat it 5 to 10 times.

When should breathing exercises be done?

The best time of day for yoga practices is twilight, early in the morning or the evening when energy fields of the body can easily respond to the quiet energy fields of nature. For the best effects, do the breathing techniques at least 15 minutes before or after yoga postures. An empty stomach is always very helpful. Drinking water during the practices is also not advised.

If twilight times are not convenient for you, breathing can be done at any time of day. Set aside a time to perform your breathing exercises and yoga routine every day.

Postures, however, must be done on an empty stomach. Wait at least two hours after eating. This is because the mind cannot be at peace. After eating, the mind is focused on digesting the food and is therefore not focused to do yoga.

At the end it suffices to say that *"Breath controls the life. Breath is the force, breath is the energy"*

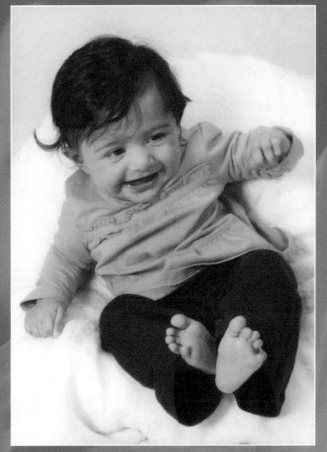

Be happy with yoga

5.11

Be healthy with yoga

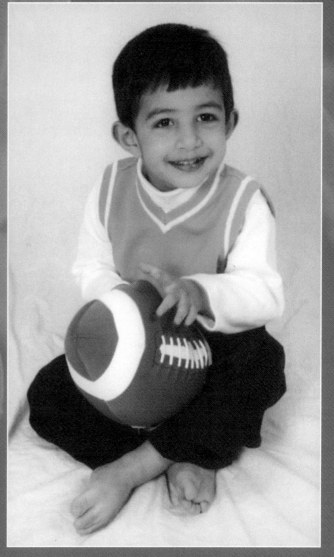

5.12

Chapter 6: Meditation

Yoga is cognitive spiritual absorption.

~ Patanjali Yoga Sutras: Chap. 1

Meditation is a very important step in yogic practices. It is the heart of yoga. One goes beyond the mind, memory and intelligence and merges with the higher consciousness, the soul.

Daily meditation practice connects you to the divine and brings bliss, joy, and contentment. Your true being is fullness, joy, and peace and not your limited body, mind or intellect. You can go beyond these with meditation.

For the pregnant woman, and for every human being, the practice of daily meditation brings inner strength, confidence, and the ability to grow as a person. It helps you to meet all kinds of situations and challenges with confidence and a clear mind. Practicing yoga will also tremendously help you during pregnancy and labor. In Ashtang Yoga, the first five stages deal with external processes, while the last three stages deal with the internal processes of the body, leading to successful progress towards meditation and Samadhi. (For a full description of Ashtang Yoga, see Chapter 1 p. 6). These last three stages are:

1. "Dharana": Holding and fixing the mind on certain points to the exclusion of all others.

2. "Dhyana": Contemplation of the self or atman (meditation).

Proper and progressive practices ease one effortlessly into meditation.

3. "Samadhi": State of super-consciousness.

6.1

"The practice of concentration on a single subject (or the use of one technique) is the best way to prevent obstacles and their accomplishments."

~ Patanjali Yoga Sutras: 1:32

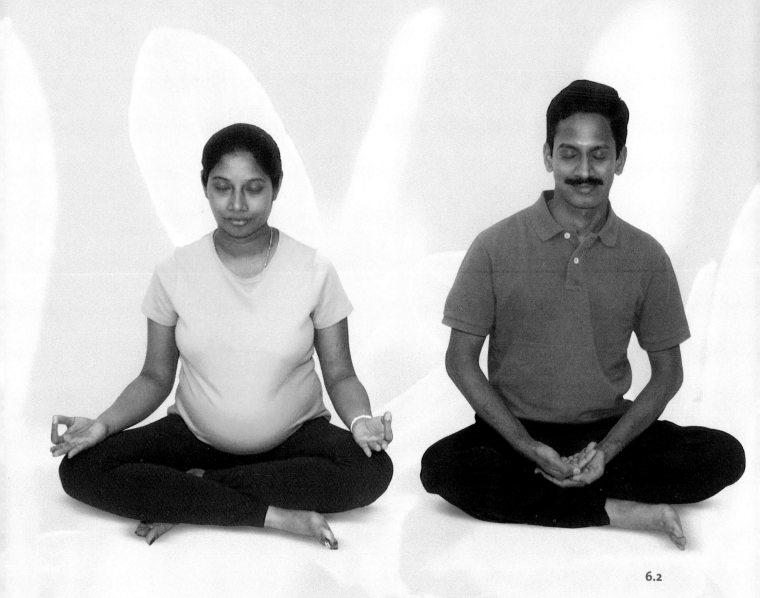

6.2

"Teach yourselves, teach everyone his/her real nature, call upon the sleeping soul and see how it awakes. Power will come, glory will come, goodness will come, purity will come, and everything that is excellent will come, when this sleeping soul is roused to self-conscious activity."

~ Swami Vivekananda

Mind is the most powerful tool to help one understand the inner world, use it and then go beyond it

In our daily lives there are constant demands; the mind is always busy, thinking of worldly affairs. This makes the mind very restless, and in due course, exhausted. The process of meditation brings a restless, chattering, cluttered, tired mind to stability, courage, confidence and focus which lead to peace, inner joy, and love. The results fill you with energy and vigor.

These processes are explained as follows:

· The normal multiplicity of thoughts in the hustle and bustle of life causes stress by mental "rush." These thoughts need to be channeled and then calmed down. (Pratyahara – withdrawal of senses)

· Yogic practices help you to sit comfortably and to move your mind from multiple thoughts to one thought. Initially this can sometimes be difficult. Try to focus on positive thought or any spiritual symbol you related to or your chosen diety – and think about its great qualities. This will bring true happiness from moment to moment. You may also want to recall a passage from scriptures or a prayer.

Lord, make me an instrument of thy peace.

Where there is hatred, let me sow love;

Where there is injury, pardon;

Where there is doubt, faith;

Where there is despair, hope;

Where there is darkness, light;

Where there is sadness, joy.

O, divine Master, grant that I may not so much seek

To be consoled as to console,

To be understood as to understand,

To be loved as to love;

For it is in giving that we receive;

It is in pardoning that we are pardoned;

It is in dying to self that we are born to eternal life.

~ St. Francis of Assisi

Stress is mental rush

The following mental attitude and thoughts will also help you:

"By cultivating attitudes of friendliness toward the happy, compassion for the unhappy, delight in the virtuous, and disregard toward the wicked, the mind-stuff retains its undisturbed calmness."

~ Patanjali Yoga Sutras: 1:33

· Begin by slowly breathing in and out. Focus on one thought (Dharna). For example, if you focus on a flame, elaborate and enjoy all of its different parts – its color, its warmth, its beauty, etc. Keep these thoughts steady in your mind.

Slowly you will learn to drop all of these thoughts and ease into meditation.

· Meditation (Dhyana) does not require an effort. It is an effortless process.

A modern mystic of India explained the process of meditation as follows:

• A mind that is fast is sick.
• A mind that is slow is sound.
• A mind that is still is divine.

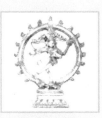
Nataraja shiva
Shiva means auspicious/good

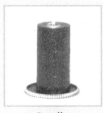
Candle

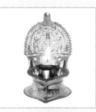
Oil lamp

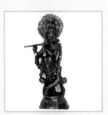
Krishna
8th incarnation in Hinduism Master of yoga

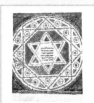
Star of David
God rules the universe in all six directions

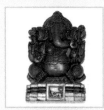
Ganeshji
Removal of obstacle

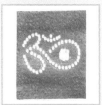
Aum
Primordial sound pious words-mantra

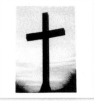
Jesus lived for others. Sacrifice is the life

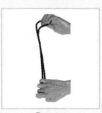
Rosary

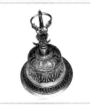
Bell

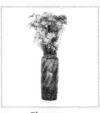
Flowers

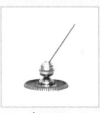
Incense

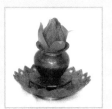
Coconut with kalash
Pot with pious water

6.3

HOW DO I BEGIN TO MEDITATE?

1. Devote 10 to 15 minutes every morning and/or evening for meditation. Try to finish important calls, work, and family obligations before beginning. You need to have freedom from these external forces and no disturbances during meditation.

2. Sit comfortably either on the floor or on a chair preferably facing east or north to benefit from the subtle effects of the earth's magnetic field. Use the same sitting mat every day.

3. Meditate in the same place every day. Choose a peaceful area of the house, which is clean and free of clutter. Do not bring food or other unclean things into the area. (You also can meditate in an office if the conditions are good.)

4. Timing: Although meditation is ideal at twilight times, it can be done at any time of the day. After all, life should be a continuous meditation with total surrendering to cosmic consciousness. It's best to meditate on an empty stomach.

5. Wear loose clothes. A leather band, leather belt, or jewelry of any kind will only obstruct the free flow of energy.

6. Sit comfortably firm on your mat but not tense with your back, neck, and head in one line for the flow of energy from the bottom of the spine to the head. Be totally relaxed. Keep a smile on your face to feel the internal relaxation and surrendering. (Meditation can also be done while sitting in a chair.)

After all, life should be a continuous meditation with total surrendering to cosmic consciousness.

7. Consider using candlelight or incense to create a soothing, pleasant atmosphere. Initially, you may want to play soothing music while learning to meditate. Eventually no external help will be necessary.

8. One of the techniques is to focus on a candlelight flame and then withdraw. Close your eyes and visualize the "flame" in the middle of your forehead between your eyebrows or in the center of your heart.

9. Associate the process with slow, deep smooth breathing in and out. Try to make the length of the outgoing breath double the incoming breath.

10. It may also be helpful to repeat certain sounds (Mantra) to help connect with your "Inner Being," although it is not mandatory.

11. Simply detach yourself from your thoughts and watch your mind go beyond it.

A new energy and vigor will travel through your body and you will feel totally relaxed, calm, fresh and full of love and surrendering to embark upon your duties.

The practices of meditation will especially help during labor, a time when you need to really focus on one thought, rhythmic breathing, and surrender.

Chapter 7: Creating a Life-Thrilling Experience with Labor

Labor is the culmination of the process of pregnancy in creating a miracle child. It is the grand finale.

It's important to understand the physiology of the process of labor and then to let nature, your instincts, and your nurse and physician work together to achieve this amazing feat.

The last three months of your pregnancy (after 28 weeks of gestation) is called the third trimester. During this time the uterus experiences contractions and relaxation activity, known as "Braxton Hicks contractions," which become more intense toward the end of pregnancy. For some women, these contractions are strong and mildly painful. The majority of women experience a feeling of hardening and a more noticeable feeling of the uterus relaxing.

The movements, positioning during labor, and general understanding of labor process should be understood and practiced ahead of time so that they become spontaneous and instinctive. If they're not practiced ahead of time, it can lead to additional stress and strain during the labor process.

General principles include:

- Relaxed breathing
- The process and understanding of focusing and calming the mind
- The attitude of surrendering
- Use of force of gravity
- If necessary, be prepared to cooperate with your physician, if an operative delivery is necessary.

In your last trimester of pregnancy, your gait also will become waddling and standing straight will be difficult. It's still important to try to stand with weight on both feet, rather than on one side and to use a wall for support whenever it is possible or necessary. During this time you should continue to do yoga's squatting poses, Pranayama breathing, and meditation.

As your pregnancy advances, certain poses may become a little difficult. Always proceed with awareness and listen to your inner intelligence to guide the body to within its capacity. Pranayama and meditation are best to be done with your partner, if possible, every day. Also try to walk outside daily. It will give you fresh energy with faith in life's natural forces and beauty.

It's also very important to know where your baby will be delivered. Visit the hospital, birthing center, or other medical facility to view its surroundings and also to learn about its philosophy. Be sure to talk with the nurses in your prenatal classes about your desire to follow the Yogic principles of labor and to have the labor process be as natural as possible. It's also important to share these details with your physician, who will help you in your method and also will help to ensure that both you and your newborn are medically safe.

"The difficulty is that a man thinks he is the doer. It is a mistake. It is the higher power which does everything and man is only a tool. If he accepts that position, he is free from trouble."

~ *Ramana Maharsi*

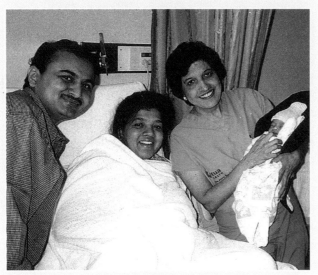

7.1 Happy Mother, Happy Father, Happy Obstetrician and a Miracle Child

Sharing the Labor Experience with Your Partner

The philosophy and practices for yoga and other natural processes should be fully understood by your partner. Throughout your pregnancy, whenever possible, he should also do asanas, Pranayama practices, and meditation with you. A couple achieving harmony and unity is a very essential part of creating a miracle child.

During your last trimester, just as practiced throughout the pregnancy, start the session with about 10 minutes of quiet breathing. This will help you tune into a deeper, more meditative state of mind. Always acknowledge the presence of your baby when practicing. It is also important during this time to be able to be silent and quiet together with your spouse. You must enjoy each other's company and share your life philosophy. This closeness will allow you to discuss the labor process without any fear and with total faith and surrender. Topics that should be discussed include: the stages of labor; the possible variations in the progress of labor; the possible variations in analgesic uses; possible variations in the techniques of delivery; episiotomy; the illumination in the delivery room; music and other calming sounds; the presence of the obstetrician; the presence of the nurse; and the presence of the neonatologist.

Joyful mother with
a miracle child

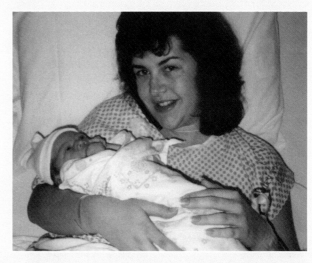

7.12

Stages of labor

First stage of labor

By definition the first stage of labor is from the onset of labor pain to the full dilation of the cervix.

At times Braxton Hicks uterine contractions are perceived as painful labor contractions. They may occur rhythmically and close enough apart (5 minutes apart or so), but they do not result in dilation of the cervix. Braxton Hicks contractions may last for several days for a short period of time, especially in the evening.

Sometimes labor starts without any warning, but most women experience a gradual build-up to real labor. Labor pains may begin at variable intervals, such as every 5 to 10 minutes, and progressively intervals come closer and pain stronger. Most delivery facilities recommend arriving at the location when pains are five minutes apart and strong for one hour. During this time a lot of slimy mucus discharge usually comes out, known as the "mucus plug," which may also be blood tinged. During this stage the cervix (mouth of the uterus) starts shortening in length from its usual one-inch in length to its paper thin length at the end of the first stage. This is known as "effacement." The cervix also softens, known as "ripening." Some women emit an involuntary clear discharge during this time. This is when the amniotic fluid that envelops the fetus during pregnancy comes out. It's called "rupture of membranes" or "water breaking." When this

occurs, you should proceed immediately to the delivering facility, even if you don't have any labor pains.

Never panic during the first stage of labor; anxiety and fear can make labor pains worse. In the very early stage of labor, when you are not sure that it is a true labor you may drink fluids in the form of clear juices, and eat soft,

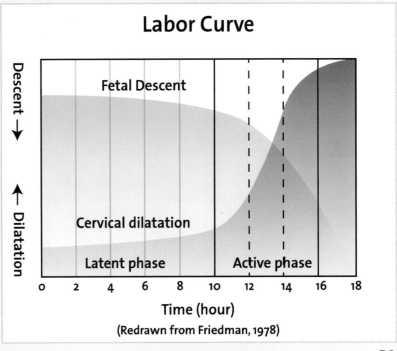

Labor Curve

Descent →

← Dilatation

Fetal Descent

Cervical dilatation

Latent phase

Active phase

0   2   4   6   8   10   12   14   16   18

Time (hour)
(Redrawn from Friedman, 1978)

7.2

easily digestible, quick calorie release simple carbohydrates until the labor contractions become rhythmic and true labor starts. Then do not eat or drink. When you get to the delivery facility, usually IV fluids will be started by your physician.

Do not start counting the intervals between contractions, unless they start coming in rapid succession, every five minutes or so. This will help to prevent exhaustion in the later part of labor, when real focusing is needed.

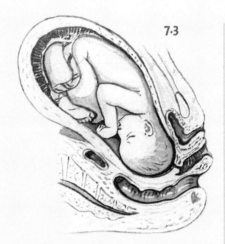

7.3

When the fetal head settles into the pelvic inlet it is called engaged. It may precede actual birth by three weeks in a primapara and a few hours to a week in a multipara.

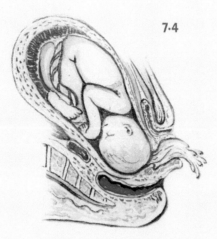

7.4

Dilatation of the cervix and rupture of membranes is some cases.

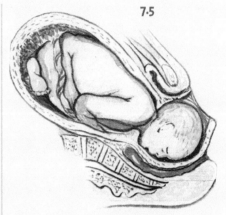

7.5

In the first stage of labor the uterus undergoes irregular or regular contractions of varying intensity. The amniotic sac (bag of waters) may or may not rupture at some point during these contractions.

Positions of Help During The First Stage of Labor

- Stand or walk while leaning against a wall during contractions, with both feet apart and grounded on the floor.
- Some women may like to be helped by their partner during contractions while standing. Breathe together and share contractions. It will be very comforting.

- Some women may like to sit comfortably on a chair with their legs spread apart, with their feet resting flat on the floor. Try leaning from the hips onto the thighs, and rock yourself back and forth forward onto soft pillows during contractions.
- If you want to lie on a bed, make sure that the head of the bed is raised to a 45-degree angle or more. This gravitational force will help in the descent of the fetus.

Second stage of labor

By definition the second stage of labor is from full dilation of the cervix to the delivery of the fetus.

The basic physiology is that once the cervix is completely open, the uterus, cervix and vagina become like one continuous column. Picture the dome of the uterus as an inverted wide open bag with the closed bottom at the top. The labor contractions then result in the descent of the fetus. As the fetus descends, its head touches the muscles of the pelvic floor. The pelvic floor muscles give rotational movement to the presenting part, bringing the back of the head (occiput) to the front of the pelvis. This is why in the majority of normal deliveries the back of the head is anterior. In some cases when the head of the fetus is relatively big compared to the cavity of the pelvis, the presenting part tries to fit into it. This results in either a transverse position of the head or a posterior position of the head. In approximately 3 to 4 percent of cases, the fetus likes to present itself with its buttocks, keeping its head in the upper part of the uterus, called breech position. As you go into further progress, comes "crowning," when the presenting part of the fetus is seen steady in the vaginal entrance. All of these different variations are known to obstetricians. But for pregnant women, it can

affect how they experience labor and how their babies will be delivered. Some mothers have big pelvises with a round shape. For these women, if the fetus is of a reasonable size, the second stage of labor is usually short and the effort required from them is minimal. Other mothers have pelvises in the shape of long in front to back diameter, with parallel pelvic sidewalls leading to a deep and narrow pelvic cavity or a flat pelvic cavity with long transverse diameter of pelvic inlet. For these women, the fetal head may have difficulty in descending. There are other mixes of pelvic make-ups that may affect delivery, but those mentioned are the most common. It's important to understand that your stages of labor will be affected by your pelvic structure, uterine force and the size of the fetus. You need to be accepting of what that is and prepare yourself to give the effort needed during this stage.

After the descent of the fetus and as crowning of the presenting part continues, the muscles at the opening of the vagina (perineal muscles) keep being stretched. During this time the obstetrician or nurse can massage and stretch these muscles gradually with mineral oil to possibly prevent the need for an episiotomy, a surgical incision through the perineum made to enlarge the vaginal opening and to assist childbirth.

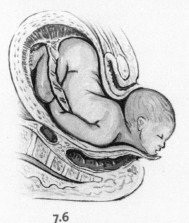

Presentation of the head. An episiotomy (surgical incision) may be needed.

7.6

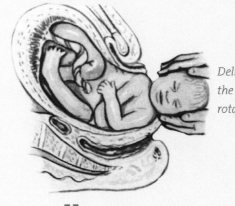

Delivery of the head and rotation.

7.7

Positions of Help During The Second Stage of Labor

The principles of gravity and energy from Mother Earth are of great value here. Some of the positions include:

- Semi-reclined position in bed (used mostly in the USA)
- If the presenting part of the fetus is not anterior, then try a left lateral position. This may help bring about the rotational movement of the fetus to bring the head from the posterior part to the anterior part of the pelvis.
- Intermittent standing squat while holding onto your knees until time of delivery.

How to Push or Bearing Down

Pushing is instinctive. When the "pain" comes from a uterine contraction, focus and gather your energy without getting tense. Take a deep, slow, long, breath and push with steady, continuous, downward force, as long as you can, using your abdominal muscles. If you've been practicing Pranayama throughout your pregnancy, the mental poise achieved will help make your pushes tremendously more effective and longer. The "awareness" during pushing should be on your pelvic floor muscles and the presenting part.

In over 40 years of delivering babies, I can say with confidence that there is a tremendous difference in the labor experience when the mother has the knowledge and mastery of this "concentration followed by relaxation" technique. Although this stage of labor is quite demanding, a woman's optimism and joy of new creation overpowers her pain and suffering.

In between pushes again use your habit of total relaxation, which you have mastered during pregnancy with meditation. This will also bring about a better "relaxation response" and improved circulation of blood to the uterus for the fetus.

Birthing Positions

Most of the birthing places and labor rooms now have "labor-delivery and recovery beds." These beds are very useful, since the mother does not have to be transferred from one bed to another during any stage of labor. The head of the bed can go up, helping the delivering mother to use the gravitational force of Mother Earth to help the fetus descend. The bottom of the bed also comes off during delivery to ensure that the delivery is as easy as possible.

Different institutions use different techniques. In my experience, lying in a semi-reclined position in a bed at a 45- degree angle or more is very effective. Squatting position can also be used successfully.

At times it may be necessary to deliver the fetus in the left lateral position. When this occurs, one of the nurses or a midwife helps with holding the upper leg, again bent at the knee.

In between pushes again use your habit of total relaxation, which you have mastered during pregnancy with meditation.

Third stage of labor

By definition, the third stage is from the delivery of the fetus to the delivery of the placenta (after birth). It usually takes a few minutes to half an hour.

The best position for this stage is semi-reclined more or less lying on the back in the bed. This helps shift the body's circulation. At times, because of blood lost during this stage, the mother may experience some dizziness. The lying position helps the body regain its balance more quickly.

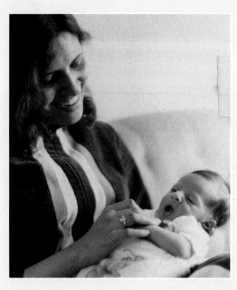

7.9

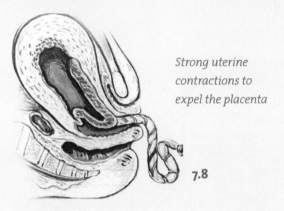

Strong uterine contractions to expel the placenta

7.8

"I saw the baby and I was lost, I was in divine love, without any words, without any mundane consciousness. "MY BABY" the Creator's greatest miracle, the most beautiful in the world."

~ Dr. Gandhi, 25th May, 1973
At her first delivery

Immediate postpartum period

Immediately after delivery, a woman is physically exhausted. But mentally, she feels accomplished, tremendously satisfied, and is filled with inner joy and thankfulness. While she holds her newborn, her faith in the cosmic consciousness, energy and divinity is reinforced.

The miracle and joy of seeing the baby makes the mother transcendental. All the pain is forgotten, and new life and optimism become reality.

It's important to bond at this time with your baby, but the length of time will vary depending upon your energy level. Usually only a few minutes are recommended to give you the necessary time to rest and recover from the strenuous process of labor. You should hold the baby while in a 45-degree upright sitting position (when you're ready) or you can bond in a lying position. Mother to baby contact is inexpressible joy. If you're up to it and have energy, you can breastfeed immediately. If you're not ready, you can breastfeed as soon as you recover from labor exhaustion.

7.10

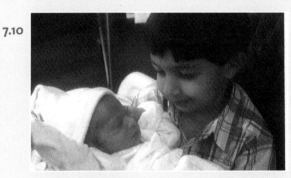

Happy sibling bonding

Pain management during labor

The word "labor" is appropriately chosen to describe the process. It definitely requires a lot of energy, both physically and mentally. Pain management during labor has become a big issue in conventional medicine. Recently, every effort is being made to make pregnant women comfortable during labor. The use of epidural anesthesia has increased markedly throughout the United States. In some institutions, it's used in 95 to 97 percent of patients. This increases comfort for the patients but raises some issues to consider.

While it's important to make the comfort of the mother a priority, it's also best to balance comfort and the medical outcome as well, in every respect. By trying to give women a "five-star experience," some doctors and nurses may overuse pain medication during labor. The early start of epidurals, especially in early first stage of labor, with heavy doses of pain medicines injected through them, is quite inappropriate. The practice can result in prolonged labor and abnormal and difficult presentations of the fetal head. Heavy epidural anesthesia may increase number of urinary catheterizations during labor, leading to the possibility of urinary tract infections, a rise in forceps delivery, more caesarean deliveries, postpartum urinary retention, and long-term backache in few cases. Pain due to uterine contractions in the first

There's a difference between "pain and suffering." Pain is a physiological, external response, while suffering is an internal, true feeling response.

stage of labor is usually very bearable, when the cervix dilates up to 3 cm or so. This is called "latent phase of labor." Subsequently, pain comes more frequently and becomes stronger and cervix dilates faster. This stage is called "active phase of labor" and usually women will require some kind of pain management, either epidural anesthesia or analgesics.

There's a difference between "pain and suffering." Pain is a physiological, external response, while suffering is an internal, true feeling response. If you are prepared to accept the process of labor and its accompanying pain, then your need for an epidural anesthesia and/or analgesics will be minimal. By minimizing the use of these medications, you will help the fetus to be fully alert at the time of delivery. You will also experience the joy of accomplishing labor on your own terms.

I am not against the joy and comforts of anesthesia and analgesics but a well prepared mother will need probably the least amount of pain medication and for a short duration. Moreover, she will be able to share in her own pain management.

You will see the face of your newborn
And instantly you will fall in love with him or her
And all your pain will be forgotten.

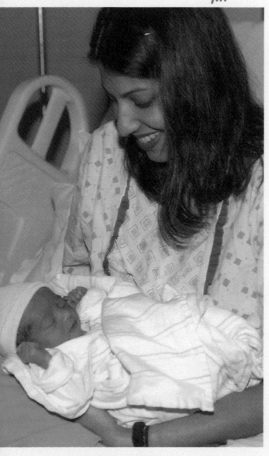

Accomplished Mother

Come Out And Play

My heart seems to beat a little faster these days.
Maybe it's the thought of my life changing in so many ways.

I've heard so many tales of sleepless nights
and tests of patience taken to new heights.

Yet my excitement grows as we count down each week
for I know soon we will finally meet.

I have a little fear I must admit,
Will I be good at it?

I daydream of baseball games and fishing trips
and passing along life's little tips.

Will you be tall? What color is your hair?
Do you like peas? What will you wear?

Can I slay the monster under your bed?
Will we be able to build a sled?

How will I explain the birds and the bees?
Oh, I must have a million of these.

Answers to questions, questions to ponder
Things to see, places to wonder

Together, we'll be the ultimate team
Limited only by what we can dream.

So as the weeks are counted down, I anxiously await
that oh - so - wonderful date.

When all of the waiting is over and done
and I can hold you in my arms, My Son.

~ Brad Lawson

(c) 1998 Brad Lawson, reprinted with the permission of the author.

Chapter 8: Yoga as Complementary Medicine to Prevent Certain Pregnancy Illnesses

Yoga has been practiced for thousands of years in Eastern parts of the world, especially in India, its place of origin, in the different forms. Available documents suggest that different types of Yoga are described in *Bhagwat Gita* (by Lord Krishna) approximately 4,000 years ago and Ashtang yoga (by Patanjali) has been practiced and written approximately 2500 years ago (around Buddha's time). In Ashtang yoga the author has described yoga very scientifically and has documented its fullest benefits. The *Patanjali Yoga Sutra* is one of the most accepted literatures for yoga in modern times.

Over the course of past 50 years, many yoga research institutes in India, the U.S., and other parts of the world have opened to provide evidence-based research to prove that yoga is a great complementary medicine for many common diseases. It not only prevents, but also helps cure hypertension, diabetes mellitus, bronchial asthma, eating disorders, and mental conditions such as depression and anxiety. A number of well- documented, case controlled studies have been published proving yoga's tremendous health benefits without any side effects (see www.svyasa.org, www.divyayoga.com, pyp.conference@gmail.com).

During pregnancy with the increase in physical and mental demands on the body, some of these diseases, such as hypertension, diabetes mellitus, and bronchial asthma, may worsen. Dangerous conditions such as toxemia or pregnancy-induced hypertension (P.I.H.), status asthmaticus (a severe episode of asthma that may threaten a person's ability to breathe altogether) and uncontrolled diabetes, low platelet count and many other life threatening diseases can be prevented largely by regular yoga practices and a yogic lifestyle, though more understanding of this science by the medical community and researchers are needed.

Studies at several well known yoga research centers in India prove that by doing yoga regularly, the pregnant woman can reduce the risk of developing complications due to these diseases. One study also found that regular yoga sessions help increase blood flow to the fetus. (see research by Svyasa, www.svyasa.org) This increased blood flow helps the fetus grow stronger physically and also has a calming effect on its mind.

The causes of toxemia or P.I.H. are still being debated. Hopefully studies will be undertaken in the U.S. and around the world to see if some of these dangerous conditions in pregnancy can be helped by a total yogic lifestyle.

Yoga and meditation also have been shown in medical studies to improve clinical depression by developing a person's inner strength. When anti-depressants alone are given without a helping hand to direct a person to yoga or other relaxation techniques, it is an incomplete therapy. Moreover, a number of documented studies have shown in India (www.svyasa.org) that when many newly-diagnosed depressed patients are taken off these medications and advised to practice yoga regularly, their mental health improves. We hope to study all these further in the U.S.

"The best health is achieved by a preventive, natural, yogic lifestyle."

Chapter 9: Yogic Diet

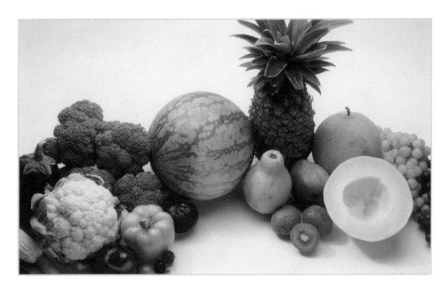

*"You are
what you eat."*

It has been said "you are what you eat." The finest portion of food nourishes the mind and as you think, so shall you be. Diet has a great influence and plays a major role in our physical well-being, energy level, and mental aptitude. It also may have an influence in preventing some of the complications of pregnancy, including toxemia or pregnancy-induced hypertension (P.I.H.). The role of appropriate diet in management of diabetes is well-known and is practiced throughout the world.

It is not only important to count the calories that you consume, but also what you eat, when you eat, and with what attitude you eat. This also includes what liquids you drink. Although lots of variations are seen in the diet of different people, but general guidelines help a lot to modify the intake of food. A yogic diet usually is a vegetarian diet but people who eat non vegetarian can also get some helpful hints in this chapter.

Yogic Philosophy of Diet

1. The foods that augment vitality, energy, strength, cheerfulness, and health are called "SATTVIKA." These foods are usually fresh, sweet in taste, and oleaginous (containing or producing oil). According to the yogic philosophy of diet, food must be prepared daily and be fresh.

2. The foods that augment anger, hurrying, and too many activities are usually bitter, sour, salty, and excessively hot. They are called "RAJASIKA."

3. The foods that make a person lazy, tired, and dull are usually stale, pungent, tasteless, sticky, overcooked, canned, and impure. They are called "TAMASIKA."

It is not only important to count the calories that you consume, but also what you eat, when you eat, and with what attitude you eat.

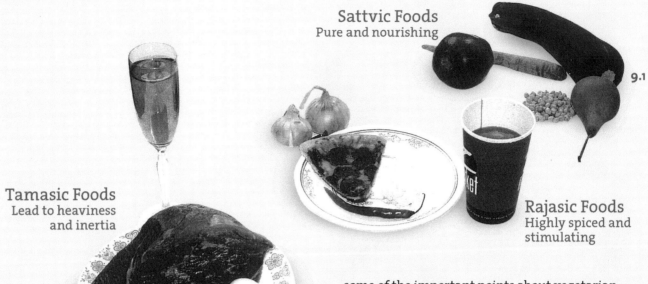

Sattvic Foods
Pure and nourishing

9.1

Tamasic Foods
Lead to heaviness
and inertia

Rajasic Foods
Highly spiced and
stimulating

When to Eat

Usually after the second trimester the appetite is more settled. The nausea reflex is gone or rarely experienced. The principle of timing for food in general is to eat only when you are hungry; but for pregnant women food should be eaten several times a day. The timing should be adjusted to accommodate your daily routines. To avoid esophageal reflux, it's always best to eat dinner early. If you have excessive nausea or vomiting during the first three months of pregnancy, then eat more frequently and in small amounts. Drinking ginger water (prepared by boiling fresh cut ginger in water for 15 minutes or so) along with honey will also help nausea. You may add fresh lemon to ginger water, if desired.

Attitude during eating

Eat with reverence to the food, with a prayerful attitude so that it makes a strong body and a healthy mind. Try to eat slowly, enjoying and relishing your food fully. This also will help in digestion. It will be appropriate to discuss here some of the important points about vegetarian and non vegetarian diets. A vegetarian diet is superior for human beings. The intestines in human beings are more than 30 feet long and have lots of folds (haustrations) which are more suitable for a vegetarian diet. In carnivorous animals the intestine is short, about 3 feet, and without haustrations, which is suitable for meat digestion. A balanced vegetarian diet helps develop a positive mental attitude and spiritual growth.

Pregnancy and Nutrition

Normally a pregnant woman requires approximately 2,400 calories daily.

Eating a healthy, balanced diet by eating a variety of healthy foods will give you all the nutrients for you and the baby. Low fat dairy products like yogurt, buttermilk, cheese, lots of fruits, vegetables, whole grains, cereals, beans and legumes can provide you with the extra calories you need.

Fluids: Drink approximately 8-10 cups of fluid. Water, 100% juices, buttermilk, low fat or regular milk etc. can be taken throughout the day.

In general, the following should be understood when following a yogic diet: Choose complex carbohydrates such as brown rice and whole wheat bread. Choose fresh fruits, and fresh fruit juices. Always choose whole grains.

In general a vegetarian diet is superior for human beings.

- Vegetarian sources of protein, such as legumes, lentils, yogurt, buttermilk and cheese are favored over non-vegetarian choices.

- Try to choose low fat options for particular foods.

- To obtain enough fiber from your diet, eat lots of fresh salads and green, leafy vegetables, bran and whole grains.

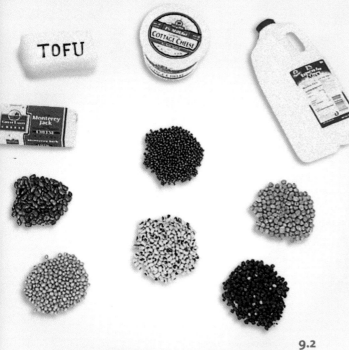

9.2

Sources of vegetarian protein

- Moong beans
- Pinto beans
- Butter beans
- Chick peas
- Green, yellow, black eyed peas
- Soya beans
- Differenct kinds of lentials

- Tofu
- Milk
- Yogurt
- Buttermilk
- Cheese
- Whole cereals (limited amount)

Daily Meal Planning Guidelines

- Eat at least 2 to 3 servings of protein.

- Eat beans, soy products, and nuts and nut butters. Eggs can also be included depending on the type of vegetarian diet you follow (or eat at least 2 to 3 servings of lean meat if you are not vegetarian).

- Eat at least 3 servings of whole grain bread, cereal, or pasta.

- Choose cereals and bread products that are fortified with iron. These, along with your prenatal vitamin, will meet you iron needs during pregnancy.

- Have at least 3 servings a day of fruit. Limit juice to 100% fruit juice.

- Eat at least 2 to 3 servings of vegetables (including at least 1 serving of dark green or orange vegetables that are high in iron and vitamin C).

- Have at least 3 servings of low fat or fat free dairy foods for adequate calcium and vitamin D intake.

See the sample menu on the next page and reference.

Recommended foods

Food Group	Amount per Day	Recommended Foods	Serving Examples
Dairy	3 cups	• Low fat yogurt • Fat free milk (skim milk) • Low fat milk (1% milk) • Reduced fat cheese or cottage cheese	• 1 cup milk • 8 ounces yogurt • 1 ½ ounces cheese • 2 ounces processed cheese • 12 ounces buttermilk
Fruits	2 cups	• Cantaloupe • Honeydew melon • Mangoes • Prunes or prune juice • Bananas • Apricots • Oranges and orange juice • Red or pink grapefruit • Avocado	• 1 cup fruit • 1 cup juice • ½ cup dried fruit
Grains	1st trimester - 6 ounces 2nd & 3rd trimesters - 8 ounces	• Fortified ready to eat cereals • Fortified cooked cereals • Wheat germ • Whole grain bread	• 1 slice bread • 1 ounce ready to eat cereal • ½ cup cooked pasta, rice, or cereal
Proteins	1st trimester - 5 ½ ounces 2nd & 3rd trimesters - 6 1/2 ounces	• Cooked dry beans and peas (such as pinto beans, soybeans, white beans lentils, kidney beans chickpeas) • Nuts and seeds (such as sunflower seeds, almonds hazelnuts, pine nuts, peanuts, and peanut butter)	• ½ ounce nuts • 1 egg • 1 tbs peanut butter
Vegetables	1st trimester - 2 ½ cups 2nd & 3rd trimesters - 3 cups	• Carrots • Sweet potatoes • Pumpkin • Spinach • Cooked green (kale, collards, turnip greens, and beet greens) • Winter Squash • Tomatoes • Red Sweet Peppers	• 1 cup raw or cooked vegetables • 1 cup vegetable juics • 2 cups raw or cooked leafy green vegetables.

Modified from American Dietetic Association

Nutrition therapy for Morning Sickness

This nutrition therapy will help you with the nausea and vomiting experienced during pregnancy.

Everyone's body is different. You may want to try the following tips to see if they work for you:

- Try to eat 6 small meals/snacks during the day. Small meals may be easier to tolerate than large meals.
- Keep easy to digest foods, such as crackers, with you during the day. You may even try eating a few crackers before getting out of bed in the morning.
- Drink water or other beverages (caffeine-free) between meals.
- Eating ginger or drinking ginger ale improves nausea.
- Lower fat foods are easier to digest. High fat foods can make nausea worse.

Recommended Foods:

You may eat any food except those on the not recommended list. Eat when you are hungry. Food without much smell may be easier for you to tolerate.

The following foods may be easier to eat:

- Cold foods such as ice cream, popsicles, or frozen fuit
- Warm foods such as mashed or baked potatoes, soups, or toast
- Spicy foods such as salsa, gingersnaps, gingerbread, or curries
- Tart/sour foods such as tomato or vegetable juice, dill pickles, lemons/lemonade, limes/limeade, or other citrus fruits
- Creamy food such as whole milk, custards, puddings, or yogurt
- Crunchy foods such as raw vegetables (particularly carrots and celery), chips, raw fruits (particularly apples or pears), nuts crackers, or dry cereal
- Soft foods such as cake, cottage cheese, cooked carrots, or green beans
- Beverages and liquid foods such as fruit juice, ginger ale, other soft drinks, water, gelatin, or broth
- Salty foods such as chips, salted top crackers, dip, pizza, or tomato or vegetable juice

Source: American Dietetic Association

The finest portion of food nourishes the mind and as you think, so shall you be.

Eating a healthy, balanced diet, with a cheerful mood will produce enough breast milk for the baby.

Breast Feeding and Nutrition

- Breastfeeding requires approximately 400 calories more than pregnancy. Eating a healthy, balanced diet, with a cheerful mood will produce enough breast milk for the baby. Breastfeeding is very important not only from the standpoint of nutrition, but also for avoidance of allergies in the baby, and the feeling of security and bonding in the newborn.

- If you feel that your baby is bothered by a certain food that you eat, stop eating that food for at least 3 days and try it again when baby is a little older.

- Drink 8-10 drinks of 8 ounces of fluid in the form of juice, milk, etc. Fluid intake is very essential to keep the adequate milk production.

- Continue prenatal vitamins, calcium, and DHA supplements as during pregnancy.

- Other important nutrients during pregnancy include:

Prenatal Vitamins

A prenatal supplement is a pill that you take daily during pregnancy. It helps make sure that you're getting the right amount of certain vitamins that are important for your baby. Ask your healthcare provider to help you choose the best one for you. Taking vitamins with diet is better tolerated and absorbed.

Folic acid

Folic acid helps in cell division and growth. It prevents certain neurological birth defects in your baby. During pregnancy, you need to take 1 mg. of folic acid every day. It's best to start taking this supplement 6 months before you start trying to conceive. All prenatal vitamins should include 1 mg of folic acid.

Iron and calcium

You also may be advised to take these supplements during pregnancy. Iron increases hemoglobin and thereby oxygen carrying capacity of blood. Calcium helps to build the bones of the fetus and helps mother during and after breastfeeding and in keeping her bones stronger.

Omega-3 (N-3)

- Omega-3 are essential fatty acids which are necessary for health. They are not directly made in our body but come from the diet.

- Eicosapentaenioc acid (EPA) and docosahoxaenoic acie (DHA) are the major n-3 fatty acids.

- The body can make EPA and DHA from alpha linolenic acid (ALA).

- Why you should get enough omega-3?

  - Needed for the development of the brain, nervous system and immune function, which is important during the growth spurt in the last trimester and after birth.

  - Adequate n-3 during pregnancy is associated with appropriate birth weight, fewer preterm births, head circumference, and cognitive development.

- Omega-3 is needed for both the mother and the baby.

- The fetus gains 50-60 mg n-3 per day during the last trimester (mostly DHA).

- The mother's stored DHA decrease by 30% after birth.

- During lactation, the mother's body loses 70-80 mg DHA per day.

- The baby can only get EPA, DHA and ALA from the mother's diet.

- Studies have found that n-3 fatty acids from the maternal diet can be found in breast milk, and in fetal cord blood.

- The recommended dose of DHA during pregnancy and lactation from either supplements or fish is 100-200 mg per day.

What are some sources of EPA and DHA and ALA (precursor of EPA and DHA)?

- Leafy green vegetables, nuts (walnuts), and vegetable oils such as canola, soy, and especially flaxseed

- Supplements

- Algae and algae oil

- Fatty fish like salmon, mackerel, trout, herring, halibut, sardines and tuna

Health is wealth and let your diet be kept optimum and ideal for you and your growing fetus.

Things to avoid during pregnancy:

- bleached products, such as those made with white flour, white sugar, white flour pasta, etc.

- caffeine (if you are used to taking tea or coffee, and have to continue, limit to 1 cup a day). Learn to prepare herbal tea or enjoy hot drinks made from boiling different spices. One of the drinks can be prepared by boiling whole or powder of cardamom, cinnamon, or clove.

- alcohol

- tobacco

- recreational and street drugs

- raw or unpasteurized milk and products from unpasteurized milk like cheese and other dairy products

- fish with high mercury levels

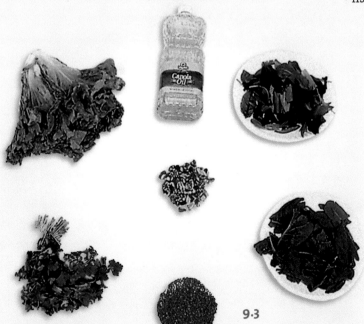

Sources of DHA

- Romaine lettuce
- Spinach
- Garden salads
- Coriander
- Leafy green vegetables
- Walnuts
- Flax seeds
- Soy seeds and canola oil

9.3

Chapter 10: Yoga and the Postpartum Period & Beyond

Pranayamas are extremely useful in reshaping your body and physiological systems

In the postpartum period, yoga will help you, the new mother, to cope with new and extra responsibility and enjoy your new creation. It will help you return to your pre-pregnancy weight and shape without any undue stress in a short time. By following a yogic diet and lifestyle, you also will be energetic and cheerful.

"After the delivery, I was always told that my life would be so different, but no one ever said how much better and fuller it would be, seeing my own creation grow every day."

First two weeks:

During this time you will need a lot of rest and emotional support. Everyone in the house should help the new mother. Chores, such as cooking, cleaning, and washing clothes, should be done by other family members to allow the new mother to adjust to her newborn. Following a good diet with increased calories and fluids (juices and milk) are essential. Adding herbs such as fenugreek (methi), Arabic gum (gunder) and carom seeds/Bishop's weed (ajwain) to foods also are useful during this time. All these are available in most Indian or Asian food stores. Deep breathing and some of the pranayamas can be started in this period.

An episiotomy or caesarean scar may be a little painful, but with the analgesic tablets given to you by your obstetrician and the seitz's bath for episiotomy, you will soon see some pain relief.

First six weeks:

All the physiological changes associated with the delivery go back to normal in six weeks. You shouldn't do any heavy exercises for the first four weeks postpartum while you are still bleeding vaginally except deep breathing, pranayama, bandhas (locks), meditation and fine joint movements (if the baby sleeps and time permits). Four to six weeks after a vaginal delivery and eight weeks after a Caesarean section, you should begin the yogic postpartum exercises described below.

Post partum breathing exercises (pranayama)

All of the breathing techniques learned during pregnancy also can be used during the postpartum period. The following additional three techniques of pranayamas are extremely useful in reshaping your body and physiological systems. Bandhas or locks are also very useful during this time. They can be started almost within two weeks of delivery.

An attitude of thankfulness and surrender is very helpful and necessary when you do deep breathing.

1. Kapal Bhati: (forceful expiration with passive inspiration)

Technique: Sit comfortably either on the floor cross legged, or in Vajrasana or kneeling position or in a chair. Keep your head, neck and back straight, firm but not tense. Breathe out fully with force by pulling the abdomen in and mimicking to blow the nose. Subsequently your breathing in or inspiration will be passive.

Repeat the expiration in quick succession. The ideal number of strokes is 60 per minute or 1 per second. Start with 1 to 2 minutes duration, increase to 5 minute. You may take breaks in between when necessary and eventually build to 15 minutes a day after six weeks.

Benefits

This increases oxygen content of every cell of the body, helps to strengthen abdominal muscles, digestion, assimilation and excretion. It tremendously helps to decrease the abdominal girth. It also helps to balance the hormones.

2. Bhastrika: (forceful inspiration and forceful expiration)

Technique: Position is the same as in Kapal Bhati described above. Take a long forceful breath in and long forceful breath out. You may raise your hands straight up dynamically with stretched open fingers while breathing in, and pull down the hands energetically with closed fists when breathing out as if you are pulling the cosmic energy in you.

The rate should be 25 to 30 times per minute. Do 15 to 20 breaths per round and do total of three rounds. Relax completely in between the rounds.

Benefits

This helps to invigorate the whole physiology, expand the lungs and tremendously increase vitality.

3. Bahya Pranayama

Technique: In a kneeling position (Vajrasana), or cross-legged sitting on the floor or in a chair, forcefully breathe out and then hold the breath for 30 seconds to 60 seconds along with pulling the abdominal wall in (Uddiyana bandha) along with the neck lock (Jalandhara bandha) and anal lock (Moola bandha). The bandhas are described in the next paragraph. Then release the neck lock by bringing the head up and release abdominal lock and the anal lock as you breathe in.

Benefits

This exercise helps a great deal in flattening your abdomen and retaining the energy in the body. Do for 3 to 5 times.

Bandhas

The Sandskrit word "Bandha" means to "hold," "tighten," or "lock." These words precisely define the physical action involved in the bandha practices and their effect on the postpartum body. The bandhas aim to lock the pranas (vital energy) in particular areas and redirect their flow into sushumna nadi (spinal cord) for the purpose of spiritual awakening.

Bandhas may be practiced individually or incorporated with mudra and pranayama practices. When combined in this way they awaken the psychic faculties and form an adjunct to higher yogic practices. They can be started almost immediately 1 to 2 weeks postpartum for a normal vaginal delivery and 3 to 4 weeks after a Caesarean section.

Moola Bandha (Anal Lock)

Sit in a comfortable cross-legged position or in the chair with the back tall and straight. Close your eyes and relax your body. Focus on your anal sphincter, perineal muscles, and the vaginal opening area. Inhale and contract these muscles. Exhale and release these muscles. Repeat 5 to 10 times and work up to 5 to 10 sets.

Benefits

The practice of mula bandha gives vigor, relieves constipation, and increases digestive fire (jatharagni) and tightens perineal muscles.

Uddiyana Bandha (Abdominal Lock)

The Sandskrit word "uddiyana" comes from the root "ut" and "did" which means "fly up." When this bandha is practiced the prana flies up through the sushumna nadi and hence the significant name.

Exhale completely through the mouth; expand the chest by a mock-inhalation movement, sucking in the relaxed abdominal muscles so that they lie flat almost in touch with the backbone. This is practiced at the end of exhalation before the beginning of inspiration. Maintain for some time and then inhale slowly.

Begin with 5 to 10 repetitions and gradually work up to 5 to 10 sets throughout the day.

Benefits

During pregnancy the abdominal muscles are stretched. This bandha helps to shorten the abdominal muscles and encourages the tissue to knit together and reach to the midline of the abdomen. When you practice this bandha, the diaphragm (the muscular portion between the thorax and abdomen) is raised up, and the abdominal muscles are drawn backwards. This bandha imparts beautiful health, strength, vigor, and vitality to the practitioner. It also prevents constipation, weak peristalsis of the intestines (the rhythmic contraction of smooth muscles to propel contents through the digestive tract) and other disorders of the alimentary canal. Uddiyana bandha also reduces fat in the belly.

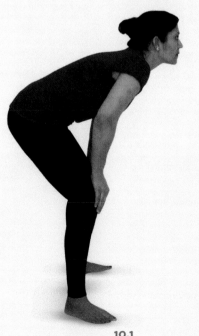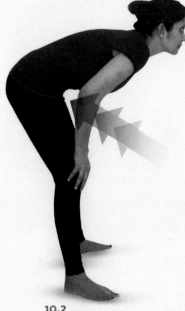

Bandha imparts beautiful health, strength, vigor, and vitality to the practitioner

10.1   10.2

Jalandhara Bandha (Glottis Lock)

This can be done either in standing or sitting position. Contract the throat; press your chin firmly against the chest at the jugular notch after inhaling. The breath is stopped at the throat. With gradual practice the pressure of air on the glottis will be released, and the whole system will be relaxed while the breath gets stopped near the throat. Hold for a few seconds – 30 seconds or so, and then bring the head up and release the breath.

Benefits

Helps thyroid function and oxygenation throughout the body.

10.3

Postpartum Yogic Asanas (Routine)

There are many yogic postures, but the most important ones for the postpartum mother are described below. All the postures done during pregnancy can also be practiced after 6 weeks of recovery, except for the pelvic widening poses, like legs wide apart in sitting and standing, which are to be avoided. Lying poses in supine position are very useful at this stage.

Added poses for postpartum period

Lying poses

1. **Leg lifting to 45º (Uttanapadasana).** Lift one leg to a 45-degree angle. Hold for 30-60 seconds or so and then bring it down slowly. Then do with alternate leg (5-10 times).

   Then repeat by lifting both legs. This asana tightens the abdominal wall and the buttock muscles.

10.4
Lifiting 45º both legs

2. **Leg lifting to 90º.** May start with alternate leg and then do with both legs.

10.5

3. **Pavan Muktasana:** First start with alternate legs and then do with both legs. Flex thigh on the hip, and flex the knee on the thigh. Then lift up your head and let your nose touch your knees as much as possible. Now try with both the legs. This is a great pose for good digestion and wind release. It also strengthens the back and pulls the abdominal muscles in. You may like to swing forward and backward on your back with both legs flexed and held, do 2-3 months after the delivery.

4. **Setubandhasana (lower back bridge pose):** Lie on your back. Keep your shoulders and head on the floor. Spread your legs about 18 inches or so apart to your pelvic width. Raise your lower back and abdomen and maintain the position as long as comfortable and then slowly bring it down. Do it several times till the optimum height of the back is achieved and you are able to maintain for a longer duration. It is great for strengthening the lower back and thighs.

5. **Naukasana (Boat position):** Lie on your back. Raise you both legs up to 45º or so, keeping your knees straight. Also raise your upper body to 45º with both hands extended in the front. (Maintain for comfortable duration for 1-2 minutes and release the pose slowly).

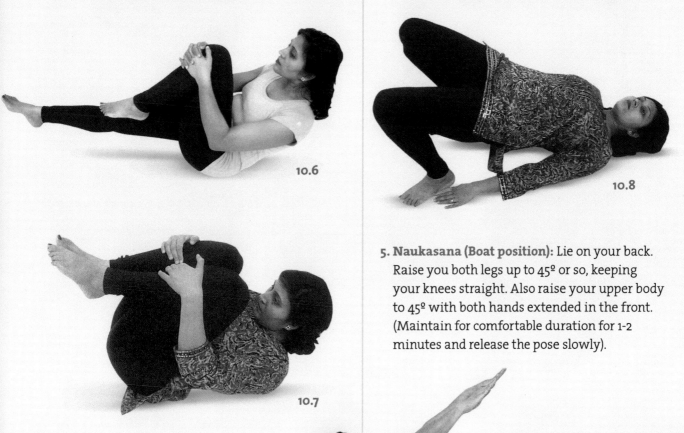

10.6

10.7

10.8

10.9

6. Adho Mukha Shwanasana (Downward-facing dog): helps back and abdominal girth.

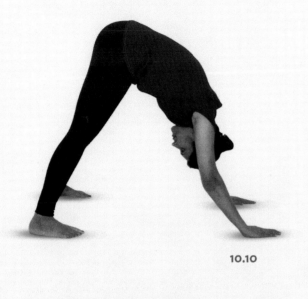

10.10

7. Shashankasana: Relaxation on your knees with extended hands in the front. (see relaxation poses (4.83)

8. Sankatasana (chair pose): strengthens knees.

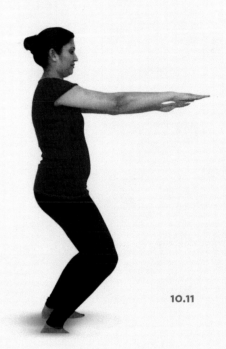

10.11

"Let over-demands of the postpartum period not bother you. Keep your faith strong, and time will pass joyfully and meaningfully."

~ *Dr. Veena S. Gandhi*

Joyful family with miracle children

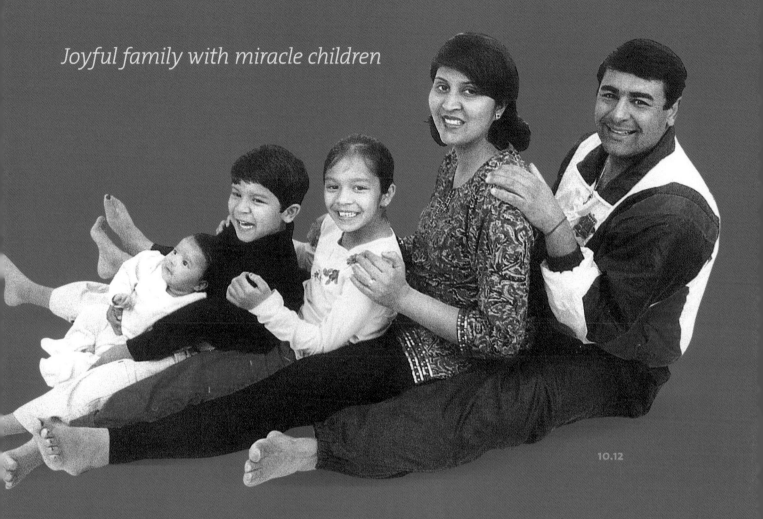

10.12

*"Let us all be active physically but calm mentally.
Let us all progress from chaos into calmness. Let us
all purify our intellect with postures, pranayama and
meditation and have meaning to our precious life."*

(OM PEACE, PEACE, PEACE)

Chapter 11:
Wisdom to Live By

To create a miracle child you and your partner must remember these important points that modern medicine has not yet addressed:

• *A deep relationship must develop between the mother and the father, not only on a physical plane, but also on a mental and spiritual plane (togetherness).*

• *For a pious soul to come as a child, the couple must surrender and have a prayerful attitude.*

• *During pregnancy the mother realizes a true synchronization with the fetal physiology.*

• *Both parents know that they have the capacity to teach during the intrauterine life.*

• *Through yoga, both parents know that they can help their child develop a positive attitude, feelings of security, and increased intelligence.*

• *Yoga improves physical comfort in pregnant women by improving their circulation and hormones and oxygen to the fetus. Yoga also helps prevent varicose veins and widens the pelvic cavity for labor.*

• *Through understanding the yogic diet and following it, a pregnant woman and her partner experience increased peace, inner perception, and balanced emotions. They also feel positive, confident and harmonized. Women who practice yoga regularly accept the natural processes of labor with ease and surrendering. They also don't need or need minimum medication or other intervention.*

• *During the postpartum period, the new mother makes an easy adjustment to her increased physical and emotional demands.*

• *Through breastfeeding, her baby receives boosted feelings of security, warmth, love, immunity.*

• *Women who practice yoga quickly return to their pre-pregnancy physiology in the postpartum period.*

Happy and healthy family units make a strong nation and the universe a better place in which to live.

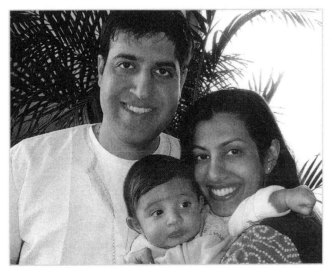

11.1

Happy, contented parents with a miracle child

Chapter 12: As Your Baby Grows

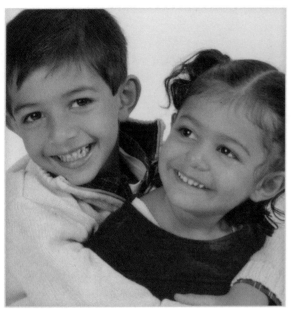

12.1

Children Learn What They Live

If children live with criticism, They learn to condemn.

If children live with hostility, They learn to fight.

If children live with ridicule, They learn to be shy.

If children live with shame, They learn to feel guilty.

If children live with tolerance, They learn to be patient.

If children live with encouragement, They learn confidence.

If children live with praise, They learn to appreciate.

If children live with fairness, They learn justice.

If children live with security, They learn to have faith.

If children live with approval, They learn to like themselves.

If children live with acceptance and friendship, They learn to find love in the world.

~Dorothy Law Nolte

As your baby grows, you will marvel in this miracle child that you and your loving husband have created. Now that the child is growing, this poem written by Dorothy Law Nolte represents beautiful thoughts to help guide you in the parenting process.

Universal Prayer

Let everyone be happy
Let everyone be healthy
Give us the strength to see good in others
Let no sorrow come to anyone

Om Shanthi, Shanthi, Shanthihi
Om peace, peace, peace

Glossary

ADHOMUKHA SHWANASANA Downward facing dog.

ANAND VALLI An important part of ancient Vedic literature, the state of joy achieved in the life is quantified.

ANANDMAYA KOSHA Bliss

ANNAMAYA KOSHA Gross Body

ANULOMA VILOMA Pranayama technique, balancing of right and left side of cerebrum. Intuitive, creative right side of brain to logical, intellectual left side of brain.

ARDHA CHAKRASANA Moon pose. Backward bend.

ARDHA-KATI CHAKRASANA Side bending.

ASANA Yogic postures for physical fitness to control the mind and ultimately be able to sit for a long duration of time for contemplation and meditation.

ASHTANG YOGA Eight limbed yoga, another name for Raja yoga, where "samadhi" is the final stage.

AUM PRANAYAMA Primordial sound pranayama, potentiated spiritual energy.

AYAMA Expanding of energy.

BADDHA KONASANA OR BHADRASANA Tailor sitting/butterfly.

BAHYA PRANAYAMA Holding the energy within by Tri Bandha in expiration hold.

BANDHAS Sanskrit word "Bandha" means to "hold," "tighten," or "lock."

BEARING DOWN In 2nd stage of labor the uterine contractions along with the personal effort by the mother to push the fetus (baby).

BHADRASANA Butterfly. Also see Baddha Konasana.

BHAKTI YOGA Path of Devotion, Kirtan and Japa, the whole universe is God's creation and so one loves each and every living and non-living thing.

BHASTRIKA Pranayama technique of forceful inspiration and forceful expiration.

BHRAMARI BREATHING Pranayama technique helps achieve intuitiveness and reach deeper existence.

BRAXTON HICKS CONTRACTIONS Painless or little painful uterine contractions in late 2nd and 3rd trimester not resulting in cervical dilatation.

BREECH PRESENTATION Type of fetal presentation when the head of the fetus is up in the fundus of uterus and buttocks or lower limbs of the fetus comes first at the delivery.

CAT STRETCH BREATHING Pranayama technique great for the back and neck.

CHAKRAS The seven energy centers in the astral body, where many nadis or astral hues come together. These chakras correspond to the nerve plexuses located in the physical body along the spine.

CROWNING Presenting part of the fetus, steadily presents at the introitus before delivery.

DEEP BREATHING Breathing with awareness, mind and total being into it.

DHARANA Holding and fixing the mind on certain points to the exclusion of all others.

DHYANA Contemplation of the self or atman (soul) (meditation).

DILATATION OF CERVIX During labor cervix dilates from 0-10 cm.

EFFACEMENT Shortening in length of cervix.

EPIDURAL ANESTHESIA Injection of medication between the spines in subdural space of spinal cord sheaths.

EPISIOTOMY Surgical incision in introitus (vaginal opening) to enlarge the opening to assist in the delivery of the fetus (newborn).

FENUGREEK SEEDS (METHI), ARABIC GUM (GUNDER), AJAWAIN (carom seeds, Bishop's weed) Spices for postpartum period, available in most Indian or Asian food stores.

FIVE MAJOR PRANAS

a. PRANA Above the umbilicus, around the heart (leads to enthusiasm, love, positive thinking).

b. APANA Below the umbilicus (perineum--anus) downward movement (responsible for excretion, negative thoughts).

c. VYANA Throughout the body (72,000 nadies or filaments of nervous system), Main Nadi: Sushumna in the middle of vertebrae, Ida on its left and Pingala on its right intertwine.

d. UDANA Around the heart, throat, palate, brain and in between. It is the upward movement of energy, last to leave at death.

e. SAMANA At naval and surrounding area, balancing Prana and apana (digestion– balancing of thoughts).

FIVE MINOR PRANAS

a. Kurma: controls eyelids and size of iris.

b. Krkala: controls sneezing and cough reflexes.

c. Devdatta: controls yawning.

d. Dhananjaya: produces phlegm.

e. Naga: relieves pressure on abdomen by belching, hiccups.

GARUDASANA (Eagle pose) Arms only.

GAU-MUKHASANA Cow pose.

GNANA Path of knowledge, logical inquiry into "Who am I?" Where will I be after death?

HATHA YOGA Yogic postures with awareness, union of "Ha", sun and "Tha", moon.

HANUMANASANA Front warrior.

IPSILATERAL Same side.

JALANDHARA BANDHA Glottis Lock. Neck lock.

JANU SIRSASANA Half angle pose.

JAPA Repetition of a mantra.

KAPAL BHATI Pranayama technique of forceful expiration and passive inspiration.

KARMA YOGA Path of action.

KRIYAS Purification exercises.

KUNDALINI YOGA Awakening of energy in the spinal column.

LABOR Process of delivery.

1st STAGE OF LABOR From the onset of labor pain to the full dilation of the cervix.

2nd STAGE OF LABOR From full dilation of the cervix to the delivery of the fetus.

3rd STAGE OF LABOR From the delivery of the fetus to the delivery of the placenta (after birth).

ACTIVE PHASE OF LABOR Strong, painful and frequent uterine contractions leading to cervical dilatation 4-10 cm.

LATENT PHASE OF LABOR Early labor, usually slow, 12-18 hours, when cervix dilates from 0-3 cm and usually labor pains are mild.

MALASANA Squatting in sitting pose.

MANTRA A mystical syllable, word or phrase helping the mind to focus during meditation. Can be repeated mentally or out loud.

MANOMAYA KOSHA Mind and emotions.

MEDITATION The state of consciousness with inner calm and stillness.

MODIFIED SARVANGASANA Half leaning against the wall with knees bent.

MODIFIED USTRASANA Camel pose.

MULA BANDHA Anus Lock.

NAUKASANA Boat pose.

NEONATOLOGY Care of newborn.

NIYAMA Contentment; internal and external cleanliness; self-study; self-restraint; and adoration of God.

OCCIPUT Back of the fetal head.

PADAHASTASANA Forward bend.

PADMASANA Lotus pose.

PANCA KOSHA Five layers of human existence.

PARIVRITA TRIKONASANA Contralateral, opposite side. Trikonasana.

PAVAN MUKTASANA Wind releasing pose.

PERINEAL MUSCLES Muscles around vaginal opening.

PRAKRITI Feminine energy.

PRANA Bio-energy, life force.

PRANAMAYA KOSHA Energy-Body/Bio-energy.

PRANAYAMA Technique to control "Prana" or vital energy.

PRATYAHARA Restraining of the senses, withdrawing from objects of desire.

PURUSHA Absolute energy.

RAJA YOGA Path of mastery over mind.

RAJASIKA DIET Foods that augment anger, rushing, and too-much activity.

RIPENING Softening of cervix.

SAMADHI State of super-consciousness, the attainment of supreme spiritual state.

SANKATASANA Chair pose. Knee strengthening.

SANSKRIT The most ancient of the human languages, often referred to as "Devanagari."

SARVANGASANA Shoulder stand.

SATVIKA DIET Foods that augment vitality, energy, strength, cheerfulness and health.

SETUBANDHASANA Bridge pose. Lower half back raise.

SHASHANKASANA Surrendering pose. Hands stretched forward.

STRESS Mental rush.

TADASANA Energy vise pose.

TAITTIRIYA UPANISHAD An important part of ancient Vedic literature, the joy achieved in life is quantified in "Anand Valli."

TAMASIKA DIET Foods that make a person lazy, tired and dull.

THREE STAGE BREATHING Complete, full breathing, leading to expansion of all 3 lobes of lungs.

TRIKONASANA Triangular pose.

UDDIYANA BANDHA Abdominal Lock.

UPAVISHTA KONASANA Sitting against the wall with legs widely stretched.

UTTANA PADASANA Legs raising to 45 degrees.

VAJRASANA Kneeling.

VEDAS The most ancient scripture in the world, scripture of "Sanatana Dharma, which is the original name for the philosophy from India. Hinduism is the name given much later.

VIRBHADRASANA Warrior pose. Lateral warrior. (front-hanumanasana).

VRIKSHASANA Tree pose.

WATER BREAKING OR RUPTURE OF MEMBRANES Involuntarily leakage of amniotic (clear) fluid through vagina.

YAMA Truthfulness; nonviolence; continence; not stealing; not collecting more than your need.

YOGA MUDRA Surrendering pose.

YOGA SUTRA OF PATANJALI The most scientific and well-known book on yoga is the *Yoga Sutras of Patanjali*, originating approximately 2500 years ago in India.

YUJ Sanskrit word, to join, leading to unity and oneness. It is the root word from which the word YOGA is derived. In spiritual terms it refers to the union of the individual to individual consciousness and individual consciousness to the universal consciousness, lower self to higher self, known as "bliss".

Bibliography

1. Yoga – Its Basis and Applications, Dr. H. R. Nagendra, 1986 – V. K. Yoga Prakashana, Bangalore, 560019.

2. Yoga – Yogasana & Pranayama for Health, Dr. P. D. Sharma, 1997.

3. "The Path to Holistic Health" – B.K. S. Ayengar, 2007

4. "Pranayama" Its philosphy and practice – Pu. Swami Ramdev, Divya Prakashan, 2006. (www.divyayoga.com)

5. Williams Obstetrics – (21st Edition, Labor Curve)

6. "Yoga – Mind & Body" – Sivananda Yoga Vedanta Center, 1998

7. Preparing for Birth with Yoga, Janet Balaskas, 1994.

8. Yoga for Pregnancy, Francoise Barbire Freedman & Daniel Hall, 1998.

9. The Sivananda Companion to Yoga, 1983. Gala Books United - London.

10. Ayureveda & the mind. The healing of consciousness - Dr. David Frowley - 1997, Lotus Press.

11. The Yoga Sutra of Patanjali - Sri Swami Satchidananda, 1978 - 2001, Integral Yoga Publications

12. The Yoga Sutra of Patanjali - with the commentary of Yvasas Bangali Baba

13. Scientific Enquiry of "Who am I"? Yogi Protoplasm, Swami Prajna Aranya

14. Swami Rama of the Himalayas - Pandit Rajmani Tigunait, Ph.D., 1998

15. Patanjali's Yoga Sutras, 2003 - Dr. H. R. Nagendra, Prof. NVC Swamy, Sri T. Mohan

Acknowledgements

To accomplish any task, there has to be first of all blessings from that super-consciousness or cosmic consciousness. I thank that energy or God for blessing me to complete this task which took more than a few years because of my busy practice and my unfamiliarity with the process of writing a book.

I acknowledge the following people, with gratitude and love, for helping me write this book:

My father, who is not with me anymore, who always encouraged me with his quiet loving blessings, and always inspired me to try new things to help people. My mother, whose blessings always flowed unconditionally, also gave me silent approval.

My Gurus, P.P. Sri Sri Ravishankarji, founder of "Art of Living" and P.P. Baba Ramdevji, founder of Patanjali Yog Pith, who have been constant sources of guidance and inspiration in my learning of yoga. They have very kindly provided me with the "forward" and "blessings" for this book. Dear Dr. Vasand Lad, has written the "Preface" for this book. I thank my guru, Dr. H. R. Nagendra for teaching me yoga. Dr. Shridhar from Bangalore encouraged me during the time when I thought I would not be able to finish the task.

My heartfelt thanks to my dear friends, Dr. Ashok Sinha and Sri Gaurang Vaishnav, who edited my book in the later stage and are my real well wishers. Similarly Christine Norris edited this book and encouraged me to publish it.

Melissa, Monica, Uma and Loretta helped me get the pictures right! I could not have pictures without their cooperation. Mrs. Charlotte Style, my office manager, is sincerely thanked for updating the manuscript.

I could not have finished this project without great cooperation from Bill Levins (Nuvonium, LLC) who rescued me by redesigning the book. I thank Mr. Bill Skinner for all his legal help and advice. I also thank the publishers who printed this book in a timely fashion. Last, but not least, my husband and my children always gave me freedom to work on whatever project I chose and helped me in all possible ways which gave me strength to grow and write this book.

About the Author

Exposed to yoga from early childhood, Veena S. Gandhi, M.D has been conducting yoga classes and organizing seminars on yoga and its philosophy for over two decades. A board-certified OB/GYN, Dr. Gandhi has over 40 years of experience in working with pregnant women and in delivering babies. Her knowledge of yoga and medical training from the Eastern and Western hemispheres gives her a unique perspective in helping couples create a miracle child.

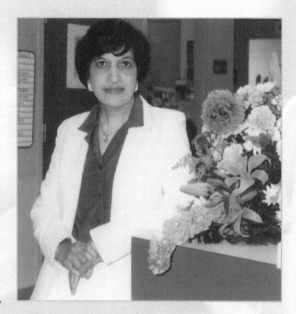

For her dedication and generosity, Dr. Gandhi has received many awards, including "Best Doctor" from the *Courier-Post* newspaper, Woman of Outstanding Achievement by the Camden County Council of Girl Scouts, and the Bhakti Visharat award for dedicated service to the community by the International Society of Krishna Consciousness. Additionally, the American Association of Physicians of Indian Origin (AAPI) awarded her the presidential award and women's leadership award for her dedicated service to AAPI.

She ran several youth programs for human values and culture. Recently she has accepted a leading position in AAPI in improving women's health. She introduced and taught yoga at every AAPI annual convention since 1995. Her latest community effort involves increasing the literacy of children in India's remote villages as a member of the Board of Directors of the Ekal Vidyalaya Foundation for the last twelve years. She was recognized for her outstanding and dedicated service to "The literacy movement" in India.

Dr. Gandhi lives in Voorhees, New Jersey with her husband, Sharad K. Gandhi. She has two grown children and two grandchildren. This is her first book.

Life is giving
Life is Love
Life is Peace

CPSIA information can be obtained
at www.ICGtesting.com
Printed in the USA
LVIC041111151212
311749LV00001B